SCREW EBOLA!

How to Protect Yourself (and your family) from a Pandemic

Wilton M. Evans

Developed in cooperation with:

Big Sky Studios, LLC,
New Mexico, USA

First Edition October 2014

Edited by: Andrew Belzer

Published by: CreateSpace Independent Publishing Platform

Author Info: Wilton M. Evans
Book Website: http://www.ScrewEbola.com

ISBN-10: 1502991535
ISBN-13: 978-1502991539

DEDICATION

This book is dedicated to all of the mentors and teachers who taught me
the difference between knowledge and wisdom.

TABLE OF CONTENTS

DISCLAIMER

It is important to note that any information found in this book is made for general educational purposes only, and is not intended as medical advice. The research and information contained within have not been approved by the FDA, CDC, or any other medical institution for the treatment of any disease.

This book is not intended to encourage you to diagnose, treat, cure, or prevent any diseases – even for lab created viruses. It is not intended to suggest that you avoid or prolong seeking professional medical care from a physician or other qualified health care professional in the event that you feel that you or someone you are caring for has been exposed to, or infected with, the Ebola virus.

Regarding the healthy body and vaccine theories discussed in this book, it is recommended that you speak to your qualified medical professional before you start, stop, or change any part of your health care program, especially if you are not sure of, or have any questions about, what is best for you or your family.

Even though I believe we have been primed for years to "report people to the authorities," for your own safety you should remain diligent and watchful of the people with whom you come in contact. It may be hard to distinguish between the flu and Ebola, but if you suspect anyone of being infected with Ebola, do not panic! Put the necessary prevention and/or isolation practices outlined in this book and other preparedness books & resources into effect. Know that you can always call 911 or the proper medical authorities if you suspect Ebola virus or any other pandemic sickness.

·

SECTION ONE – EBOLA FACTS & FICTION

It is early fall, 2014. Ebola has dominated the headlines and is all the fear for some people right now. Americans listened to the news reports on what was happening in Africa as Ebola spread to pandemic proportions. Many did not even believe that it would hit American territory, while others knew it was only a matter of time.

Authorities told everyone to relax as the virus would not spread to other countries. They reassured worrying minds by saying there was no way that we here in the United States would ever face the disastrous results that Africa has experienced. And then, shortly thereafter it was announced that the first case within the United States has been confirmed, right here in Dallas, Texas; inside the borders of the USA. Just a few days later another case was announced.

While our government and health authorities might have been initially semi-passive about Ebola, you need to be proactive. The lack of good, true information in the face of all the sensationalist fear-mongering is what bothers me most. Disinformation is spreading faster than Ebola.

I am not a medical doctor. I have a biology and psychology degree. I am a researcher, wellness advocate, and I'm pro humanity. I have children. I want to see humanity continue. I have a good grasp on the human body and specialize in turning to nature to make our bodies strong, especially in the face of pandemics. I've never been one to shy away from frightening situations.

Even though I am not a doctor it does not mean that you can't learn something from me. I have researched medical journals as well as the history of how the various strains of Ebola have effectively been dealt with in the past. I'm being proactive, and I am out there helping other people. Like I said, I want to see humanity continue.

My goal is not to instill fear but rather educate and give you information based on my research and understanding of how the human body works and functions. You need to educate yourself about Ebola so that you can protect yourself and your family. Don't wait for the government or "authorities" to take care of you. There has never been a time in history that allowing a system to take care of you has ever provided a "happily ever after." If you want to win the battle against anything in life, you need to step up to the plate, be informed, and take the appropriate steps.

For ongoing updates, vaccine detox protocols, resource guides, and homemade vaccine techniques and documentation, visit:

www.ScrewEbola.com

Having a strong immune system and avoiding needles are two of the best ways to be successful in the fight against Ebola. Few people, including scientists, understand fully how the virus does what it does and how it harmonizes itself with both nature and living organisms. We've been mostly isolated from pandemics here in the United States, and our news is highly censored (regardless of what you've been taught). The majority of people have no idea what this Ebola strain is capable of.

Ebola History – A Brief Overview
Ebola is part of the Filoviridae classification. It is a virus that has a threadlike structure ("filum" in Latin means "threadlike"). It was given its name due to the location of the first identified outbreak in the 1976, the Ebola River in Zaire. To date, the Ebola virus has been shown to be self-limiting as it has typically died out quickly. However, this time is different. It has now become known as the Ebola crisis due to the

number of deaths the outbreak has caused and the number of countries that have diagnosed infections.

Not much is truly known about Filoviridae virus strains in the medical community. There is likely a natural 'reservoir' host of the virus, but it has not yet been completely identified. Bats, monkeys, apes, and other jungle creatures are the likely source, but no definitive host has been determined because this strain seemingly came out of nowhere.

Previous to this outbreak, there were 5 previously typed Ebola subtypes, which may all be different viruses with different generational mutations. Being a virus, any strain of Ebola needs a host to live, survive, and replicate. It is believed that the initial infection of an outbreak occurs through contact with an infected animal.

The First Outbreaks
The very first Filoviridae outbreak happened in Germany in 1967 where lab workers became infected by a strain called 'Marburg,' named after Marburg, Germany, the site of one of the outbreaks. The virus was carried by green monkeys that had recently come from Uganda. In this breakout, 31 people were infected and 7 died for a 23% fatality rate. Only one generation of the outbreak occurred. It was quickly contained but not without residual fear in the scientific community. There were no further Marburg outbreaks until 1975, when only a few people were exposed and infected.[1]

Ebola was the second Filovirus to cause an outbreak, the first happening in 1976. Many of the medical centers closed down due to the quick spread of the hemorrhagic virus. Many in the medical field died. As stated earlier, this became known as the Zaire Ebola strain due to the location of the outbreak. Villages were quarantined which quickly controlled the spreading of the outbreak. And so, researchers quickly lost interest after the virus faded. Not much was discovered or known about this strain.

In 1989 monkeys in a primate facility in Virginia were found to be

---

1 For a chronological table of outbreaks of the Marburg virus, visit http://www.cdc.gov/vhf/marburg/resources/outbreak-table.html

infected with Ebola. Through 1989-1992 and again in 1996, other facilities faced the same reoccurring issue. This strain was from Asia but did not appear to have a great affinity for infecting humans.

Back to Africa in 1994-1996: 5 different areas were confirmed to have two subtypes of active Ebola. In 1994, a scientist from Switzerland became infected and was transferred back to Switzerland for care. This became the best study for human Ebola infection.

In 1995, the Ebola outbreak became news and attracted widespread attention for the first time, generating further interest in studying Ebola. Blood transfusions began to cut the mortality rate. It was identified that antibodies were not the cause of the increased survival, but rather increased white blood cells, platelets, erythrocytes and blood co-factors were likely the basis for recovery.[2] Essentially, this means *that the immune system of the patient* was stimulated, causing the person to recover. Antibodies didn't help. It was bolstering the natural disease-fighting system of the human body that made the difference.

It was also noted from follow-up testing of patients that had Ebola that people who had previously compromised immune systems before contracting the virus seemed to carry the Ebola virus, antigens, or genomes much longer.

Airborne or Not?

With the ability to study Ebola more effectively during the 1994-1996 outbreaks, the only observation regarding control of the virus was that seemed to be somewhat reliable was that transmission occurred routinely in households, between family members. This led to the belief that exposure happens during close contact and exposure to bodily fluids. The rainy season, harsh jungle conditions, and other environmental factors (such as difficulty of travel to remote areas) wrecked the ability to accurately research Ebola in the wild.

However, none of this ruled out the possibility that Ebola was also spread through airborne transmission. [3]

---

2 http://jid.oxfordjournals.org/content/179/Supplement_1/ix.long#ref-97

3 Johnson E, J. N. (1995). Lethal experimental infections of rhesus monkeys by aerosolized Ebola virus. Int J Exp Pathol.

It was further noted that with the ability to study the1989 outbreak in a controlled environment, there was an airborne pattern that was detected, as well as higher concentrations of the virus found in the nose and lungs. This suggested the virus was indeed airborne. [4]

The eyes and mouth were most common routes of receptivity. Mucous membrane exposure, exposure through cuts in the skin, and swallowing was cited as ways the virus entered the body.

It also appears that the more ill a patient is the more viral Ebola becomes.[5] It can take anywhere from 2 to 21 days before a person exposed to Ebola becomes sick.

Aggressive and Intelligent

There appears to be a glycoprotein that goes along with this virus. This glycoprotein serves as a decoy so that the immune system is not effectively alerted. The Ebola virus also appears to attack the spleen and lymph nodes which additionally shuts down the immune system. Your immune system is your defense against Ebola.

Here we have a very aggressive and intelligent virus that causes a lot of damage to the body without the help of the immune system.

To this day, little is understood about Ebola genes. The virus has less than 12 genes but still is able to manage itself, replicate, and infect humans. With the few genes it contains, this virus remains a mystery to scientists. It has shown to be resistant to many modern pharmaceutical anti-viral drugs but no one knows exactly how that is done. There is speculation that the Ebola virus can mess with genes and double-stranded RNA inside cells.[6]

---

4 A) Peters CJ, Johnson ED, Jahrling PB, et al. Filoviruses. In: Morse S, editor. Emerging viruses. New York: Oxford University Press; 1991. p. 159-75; and B) Jahrling PB, Geisbert TW, Jaax NK, Hanes MA, Ksiazek TG, Peters CJ. Experimental infection of cynomolgus macaques with Ebola-Reston filoviruses from the 1989–1990 US epizootic. Arch Virol Suppl 1996;11:115-34.

5 Dowell SF, M. R. (1999). Transmission of Ebola hemorrhagic fever: a study of risk factors in family members. J Infect Dis.

6 Harcourt BH, Sanchez A, Offerman MK. Ebola virus inhibits induction of genes by double-stranded RNA in endothelial cells. Virology 1999. (in press).

More Texas Outbreaks

It is also interesting to note that there have been 2 prior Ebola infections in Texas. Both were related to the Hazleton's Texas Primate Center in Alice, Texas. These were with a virus strain, Ebola-Reston, which usually does not infect humans. However, after exposure to infected monkeys at the Hazleton's Primate Center in Reston, Virginia in November of 1989, one of blood tests on a monkey handler showed antibodies. This indicated that this handler had been exposed in the past. [7] (NOTE: Only one of these infections is included on the CDC chronological list [below], and they do not show that the handler tested positive).

To date, there have been only 33 outbreaks of Ebola infections, with 26 of those affecting far fewer than 100 people. The largest previous outbreak infected a total of 425 people.

Compare that to the current outbreak, during which close to 5,000 people have died from the virus out of the nearly 10,000 infections reported to date (mid-October, 2014).

This in no way is a complete documentation of all the Ebola outbreaks through the years. I just chose to outline the documented beginnings of each viral strain.[8]

Something that is widely talked about on the internet is that if the Ebola virus is truly not airborne, cannot exist outside the body, and can only be transmitted through bodily fluids, then why the need for total head-to-toe protection? The respirator masks are serious business and filter out viruses. Pictures show the cleanup crew in full hazmat suits cleaning up the Dallas apartment in which Thomas Eric Duncan had been staying before his diagnosis. The clean-up occurred a full four days after the man was diagnosed. Overkill? Or do they know something that hasn't been widely publicized yet?

---

7 https://web.stanford.edu/group/virus/filo/ebor.html

8 For a table of known and documented Ebola outbreaks to date, visit:

http://www.cdc.gov/vhf/ebola/outbreaks/history/chronology.html

Symptoms of Ebola

Now that it is autumn, we are starting the flu season. This makes Ebola even more frightening because the symptoms often mimic the flu: headache, dry, sore throat, stomach ache, and body aches. If people have Ebola, they could very well be walking around thinking they simply have the flu.

Most people do not run to the doctor when they get the first signs of the flu. Obama Care and the exorbitant cost of today's health care will also cause people to put off going to the doctor. People will truly not know if they are walking around with the flu or with something much worse. They are also contagious as well.

As the symptoms worsen, just like with the bad flu strains, you may feel very tired and weak. You will have nausea, diarrhea and vomiting. Your temperature begins to rise and you experience stomach pain and more nausea. You will probably see the typical Ebola tongue within a few days of having a fever. Your tongue will be white, furred, with a bright red center.

These symptoms sound just like the flu over the past couple of years, doesn't it? How many people do you think want to run to the doctor, just to be put into isolation for several weeks and be extremely scared? Not many.

I've said it once and I'll say it many times, we have learned to turn a blind eye to what we don't want to deal with. We are a culture that needs escapes from reality instead of dealing with the stark truth.

The virus begins to invade and kill the cells in your body. It has invaded your gastrointestinal tract, spleen, liver and adrenal glands. Clotting is compromised because your liver is decomposing. You will either bleed easily or your blood will turn jello-like inside your veins. Swelling occurs in various parts of the body as organs are invaded. Rashes on the body, hiccups, loss of appetite and red eyes can occur. Your mouth begins to be covered in sores and eating is not possible. The virus is so swift moving that your organs will break down and your blood pressure drops dangerously low.

The Critical Window

There is usually a short window of a couple days where people begin to feel better and clinically show improvement. There is only a 30% cure rate so after these couple days, the symptoms may worsen quickly.

As the symptoms worsen, people will become very scared. Internal bleeding that flows out of the body's orifices can occur, but does not happen in a small percentage of cases. Your skin begins to break down and every tiny injury turns into the horrible pictures we have all seen. Death usually happens between 6-16 days after symptoms appear. The pain is unbearable.

A New Strain of Ebola?

This Ebola outbreak was originally reported to be the Zaire strain, by far the deadliest to this point, having a mortality rate near 90%[9]. The symptoms appear to be identical to previous Zaire Ebola outbreaks, but this new virus appears to be more difficult to control.[10] The CDC states this current virus is around 97% the same.

This new strain is tentatively being called the Guinean Ebola Virus ("EBOV)[11] but mostly it is still being referred to as the Zaire EBOV. Just know that we are dealing with a different strain so the health officials and the government cannot 100% accurately predict the future regarding patterns of infection and progression of the disease.

I'm not trying to scare you; I am trying to impress upon you exactly what we are dealing with so you can take preventative action. Fear is worse than Ebola ever will be. Fear is also deadlier than any virus can ever be. Keep a level head about Ebola. It is something to be alert and proactive about, but fear paralyzes and often causes people to make mistakes they normally wouldn't make.

---

9 There appear to be a few polymorphisms at "positions 2124 (G→A, synonymous), 2185 (A→G, NP552 glycine→glutamic acid), 2931 (A→G, synonymous), 4340 (C→T, synonymous), 6909 (A→T, sGP291 arginine→tryptophan), and 9923 (T→C, synonymous)" which make this strain different.

10 Dudas G, Rambaut A. Phylogenetic Analysis of Guinea 2014 EBOV Ebolavirus Outbreak. PLOS Currents Outbreaks. 2014 May 2. Edition 1. doi: 10.1371/currents.outbreaks.84eefe5ce43ec9dc0bf0670f7b8b417d.

11 Sylvain Baize, Ph.D., Delphine Pannetier, Ph.D., Pharm.D., Lisa Oestereich, M.Sc., Toni Rieger, Ph.D., et al. Emergence of Zaire Ebola Virus Disease in Guinea. The New England Journal of Medicine. 2014

The Truth About How Ebola Is Spread

As the documentation above shows, Ebola is not only spread through bodily fluids. We are not yet being told the truth about this, but the truth is out there if you dig for it. The fact is there are several ways you can contract the Ebola virus.[12]

The number one way that the Ebola virus spreads is through direct person-to-person contact.[13]

The virus can still be found in semen for up to 91 days after the first symptoms. This means that even though Ebola is cleared from the blood, it can still be found in certain parts of the body, like gonads, mammary glands, and the eyes. Therefore, Ebola can be transmitted through sexual activity long after someone is cured. According to the World Health Organization ("WHO"), the Ebola virus has also been detected in urine and in breast milk.[14]

Ebola is not yet officially classified as an airborne virus (like SARS or the flu) since its main mode of transmission is believed to be through direct inter-human contact. That does not rule out the fact that the aerosol (airborne) aspect of Ebola can and does infect people. Ebola easily becomes airborne when it is included with the body fluids of a sneeze, vomit, diarrhea, or coughing. It takes as little as 1-10 tiny aerosol organisms to infect a person with a viral hemorrhagic fever like Ebola. One tiny drop lands on your hand, you rub your eyes and you are now infected. It's that easy. In fact, the WHO finally admitted this in October 2014 (see footnote 13).

A Wider Pathogenic Footprint

Add to this fact that a recent study at MIT proves that the pathogenic footprint (i.e. how far infective agents travel) is up to 200 times further for coughs and sneezes than previously thought.[15]

---

12 Rowe AK, Bertolli J, Khan AS, et al. Clinical, virologic, and immunologic follow-up of convalescent Ebola hemorrhagic fever patients and their household contacts, Kikwit, Democratic Republic of the Congo. Commission de Lutte contre les Epidemies à Kikwit. J Infect Dis 1999;179((Suppl 1)):S28-35.

13 Franz, D. R., Jahrling, P. B., Friedlander, A. M., McClain, D. J., Hoover, D. L., Bryne, W. R., Pavlin, J. A., Christopher, G. W., & Eitzen, E. M. (1997). Clinical recognition and management of patients exposed to biological warfare agents. Jama, 278(5), 399-411.

14 http://www.washingtonpost.com/news/to-your-health/wp/2014/10/08/sex-in-a-time-of-ebola/

To give you an idea of how Ebola can be airborne, look at the flu. It is considered an airborne transmission virus, and people catch it like wildfire. Why are these considered airborne transmission diseases? It is the fluid (or droplets of body fluid) that becomes airborne through a cough or sneeze, and then causes infection in others.

A sneeze exits the mouth at up to 100 mile per hour, and a single sneeze can expel up to 100,000 germs into the air.[16] Why would this be any different with Ebola? This is what transmission through contact truly means. Ebola could very well be transmitted as easily as the common cold or flu, but, based on history, Ebola will kill 50-90% of all people that become infected.

Lack of Hygiene

I am really irritated by the lack of hygiene I see people have out in public. The reason I am so easily irritated is the selfishness people openly display. There is a ripple effect to lack of hygiene that many people are too self-absorbed to see. I see people blow their nose in restaurants, sneeze and cough very loudly and forcibly (mostly without covering their mouth), pick their nose, fail to wash their hands after going in a public bathroom, or spit. That's just what I see; I am sure there is much more that goes on than just that.

The CDC was finally forced to admit that a sneeze or a cough could transmit the disease.

Tom Frieden admitted on October 7, 2014 "That is not to say it's impossible that it could change [to become airborne]," he continued. "That would be the worst case scenario. We would know that by looking at… what is happening in Africa…"[17]

Again, this came after months of vehemently denying that Ebola could be passed on through any means other than direct contact.

---

15 http://newsoffice.mit.edu/2014/coughs-and-sneezes-float-farther-you-think

16 http://www.webmd.com/allergies/features/11-surprising-sneezing-facts

17 Viebeck, E. CDC: Airborne Ebola possible but unlikely. The Hill. 2014

Foodborne Transmission

Another consideration that has sparked interest and concern is the chance of foodborne transmission.[18] Pigs, when injected with Ebola, showed various signs of the disease and quick transmission to other pigs.[19] If the pigs were slaughtered with the virus, there is a chance that transmission of Ebola could come from humans eating meat from tainted pigs or other virus-carrying animals like monkeys, deer, bats, and other types of "bush meat." In fact, this is one of the theories about how the virus first spread to and manifested in humans; the consumption of bush meat.

Pigs and Pets

As in the scenario of the pigs, family pets have shown to also become infected with Ebola.[20] Ebola can transfer from human to animal and animal to human. How many people let their dog eat off their plate? Or allow their animal to snuggle in with them in bed? Or lick their face and mouth? Yes, pets are often considered to be one of the family. Nothing wrong with that, but these are scenarios in which Ebola can spread.[21]

A dog in Madrid, Spain was euthanized by court order because it had been exposed to Ebola. Excalibur, the Ebola dog, was a pet to the nurse assistant that had contracted the disease.[22]

Spreading Through Fomites

Infected surfaces are another form of Ebola transmission. Ebola does not die with the body of human or animal. It remains active in the blood and organs after death.

While transmission through contaminated surfaces is low, it still occurs.

---

18 Bausch DG. Ebola virus has a foodborne pathogen? Cause for consideration, not panic. J Infect Dis 2011; early online publication May 12

19 Kobinger GP, Leung A, Neufeld J, et al. Replication, pathogenicity, shedding, and transmission of Zaire ebolavirus in pigs. J Infect Dis 2011; early online publication May 12

20 Allela, L., Bourry, O., Pouillot, R., Délicat, A., Yaba, P., Kumulungui, B., Rouquet, P., Gonzalez, J-P., & Leroy, E. M. (2005). Ebola virus antibody prevalence in dogs and human risk. Emerg Infect Dis, 11(3), 385-90.

21 Acha, P. N., & Szyfres, B. (2003). In Pan American Health Organization (Ed.), Zoonoses and Communicable Diseases Common to Man and Animals (3rd ed., pp. 142-145). Washington D.C.: Pan American Health Organization.

22 Durden, T. Us Ebola-Fighting Troops Mission Could Last A Year; Spain Quarantines 6, Euthanizes Dog; US Patients Conditions Worsen. ZeroHedge.com. 2014

The amount of the time that Ebola can survive outside the body depends on the fluid, temperature, humidity, and light source.

Ebola survives the longest around 37 degrees Fahrenheit, under low light and around 37% humidity. A study done in Russia found that the Marburg virus (Ebola's 'cousin') could survive up to 4 -5 days on contaminated surfaces, but in aerosol it was not stable and survived only a few seconds.

There is not a lot of research done on infective surfaces. The one document that is quoted the most often states that Ebola "was not found" in tests done on surfaces in an isolation unit. However, at the end of the paper, it was disclosed that they had continually disinfected the room with known Ebola virus killers so that may be why no virus was detected.[23] Really? That is the basis for stating the virus can't survive on different surfaces? I guess not, if you're spraying the surfaces down frequently.

Fomite is a word we hear a lot when talking about transmission. A fomite is any surface that can be contaminated and carry the virus. This would include surfaces like: furniture, clothes, utensils, toilet seats, soap, even skin and hair. Viruses in dried blood have been shown to have the longest life on a fomite surface. The virus is still present and infectious for 4-5 days, possibly longer.[24]

If you touch something that has been infected and then eat something, that contamination could be enough to infect you. The virus will replicate itself more than a million times each day. Even if you are not aware that you have Ebola, you can pass the virus onto others, despite what you are told. Once it enters your body, the virus will attempt to replicate itself and invade every part of your body.

If you shouldn't be concerned about catching the Ebola virus, have you ever wondered why you are seeing pictures of workers wearing full body hazmat suits with respirator masks? Ebola is a level 4 biohazard,

---

23 Baush, D.G., Towner, J.S., Dowell, S.F., Kaducu, F., Lukwiya, M., Sanchez, A., Nichol, S.T., Ksiazek, T.G., Rollin, P.E. (2007) Assessment of the Risk of Ebola virus Transmission from Bodily Fluids and Fomites. JID. 196 (Suppl 2)

24Ryan Sinclair, Stephanie A. Boone, David Greenberg, Paul Keim and Charles P. Gerba. Persistence of Category A Select Agents in the Environment. Applied and Environmental Microbiology, 2007

which is the most dangerous level that is assigned to biosafety. To put this into perspective, rubber gloves are all that you need when dealing with AIDS. A basic mask will prevent transmission of Tuberculosis, but the Ebola virus needs total body coverage for protection?

Transmission by Insects

Lastly, let's discuss insects as a mode of transmission. We are nearing the end of mosquito season, but in Southern states like Texas, we can see mosquitoes hanging around throughout the winter if it is a mild one.

Ebola is part of the Rhabdoviridae family of viruses, which have a negative strand RNA genome. Insects are able to transmit Rhabdoviruses by horizontal transmission.[25] This means a disease is passed to other individuals of the same species that are not in a parent-child relationship This is an important aspect to consider regarding transmission because the Ebola outbreak in Alice, Texas showed that Ebola was passed on to other monkeys by horizontal transmission, not vertical transmission (from parent to child).[26]

Mosquitoes are only a small concern. Bedbug, flea, and mite infestations have almost grown to near-pandemic proportions in some areas. Using common sense, if an insect consumes human blood and then moves to another human for another blood meal, what could happen? Bedbugs are not thought to be a vector in the transmission of blood-borne diseases, other than Hepatitis-B. Fleas, ticks, and mites, however, have been shown to transmit various diseases, including various types of plague. It could be a very real possibility that not only mosquitoes, but any insect that feeds on blood (mites, bedbugs, ticks, etc.) could also transmit the Ebola virus, although no specific research has yet been done.

With all that being said, it appears that the most infectious times are when someone has full-fledged Ebola symptoms. The beginning stages of Ebola do not exhibit the easy transmission that the later stages have.

25 Ryusei Kuwata, Haruhiko Isawa, Keita Hoshino, Yoshio Tsuda, et al., RNA Splicing in a New Rhabdovirus from Culex Mosquitoes, Journal of Virology 2011

26 Waterman, T. Ebola Reston Outbreaks. Stanford University, 1999

SECTION TWO – RESISTANCE: HOW TO TURN YOUR BODY INTO A FORTRESS

It doesn't make sense to focus only on how to deal with Ebola once you have it. It is my belief that we can quite possibly prevent Ebola from ever taking hold in the body in the first place. This may or may not be valid. However, look at the facts. Even with how contagious Ebola can be, not everyone in Africa has become sick from the virus.

History has shown that only 30% of doctors died that had worked with Ebola when the Zaire strain was first discovered. Even though others were exposed, many did not get the virus. No one can say for sure why some did not get sick with Ebola, but much research points to a healthy immune system as a primary means of protection.

The Immune System Factor

Your immune system is your key to survival. I can't remember where I read it so I cannot give documentation, but someone working with Ebola had written that they could begin to predict in Africa who would die or who would live when they came in to the hospital infected with Ebola. If the person was in the beginning stages and their immune system was sufficiently stimulated, they ended up being a survivor.

On a similar note, Dr. Erica Ollmann Saphire Ph.D., (Professor, Department of Immunology and Microbial Science, The Scripps Research Institute) on a YouTube presentation talked about the role of the innate health of the immune system and survival.[27] To prepare your body to be naturally strong against all invaders and enemies, you must focus on your immune system.

Additionally, Ebola has shown to cause major CD4 T-cell death. There are natural remedies you can take that will strengthen, stimulate or protect the CD4-T cells.[28]

Simple Ways to Strengthen Your Immune System
Here are a few basic steps you can take to build up your immune system:

Juicing: Juicing, while often considered to be a fad diet, is actually one of the most potent ways to get mega doses of nutrition into your cells very quickly. You cannot get this much easily-absorbable nutrition from any supplements. Start juicing every day. Even if you begin with 1fresh, raw juice a day, your body will begin to be flooded with raw nutrition. Having a strong body with nutrient-dense intake creates a strong immune system. You can get free juicing recipes off the internet, from my website, and even on my Facebook page.

Get outside. Some people claim UV light will kill Ebola, while others deny that normal UV from sunlight can damage the virus. Either way, sunlight boosts your immune system and helps your body to make its own vitamins, especially Vitamin D (the "sunshine" vitamin). This is important. While you are outside daily, do something. Move your body; whether it is gardening, walking, or dancing around like Michael Jackson. Find something to do to move for at least an hour every day. Do NOT wear sunscreen as this will inhibit the production of Vitamin D from sunlight.

The Lymph System – A Major Factor
Your immune system and lymphatic system are closely tied together. You will not have an impenetrable immune system if your lymphatic system is compromised. Ebola directly attacks your lymphatic system as one of its first de-arming measures.[29]

27https://www.youtube.com/watch?feature=player_embedded&v=H8IFC8GQvNE#t=15m30s

28 Manisha Gupta,, Christina Spiropoulou, Pierre E. Rollin,. Ebola virus infection of human PBMCs causes massive death of macrophages, CD4 and CD8 T cell sub-populations in vitr. Virology. 2007

29 Waterman, T. Ebola Tissue Tropism and Pathogenesis. Stanford University, 1999

Your lymphatic system is the largest circulatory system in your body. It is twice as big as your arterial blood supply system.

Your lymph is like the drains in your home. Your toilet, sinks, bathtubs, shower, and washing machine all have drains. The drainage system of your body; your lymph system is exactly like the drainage system in your house.

Clean up your lymph system.

In this analogy, the faucets in your house, the pipes that bring water to your house, are your blood supply. What happens if the drainage for your toilet becomes clogged? Waste is backed up and goes all over your floor, right? This is the same thing when your lymph becomes backed up. Your home must maintain a clear exit so that the wastes don't remain inside. Just as your house needs to keep drainage pipes clear, your body needs to have a properly working lymph system in order to remove wastes effectively.

We hear so much about blood, blood, blood and the cardiovascular system, cholesterol in your blood, blood platelets, etc. yet we rarely hear about the lymph system. However, your lymph system is THE most important part of your body's immune system. If there was a hierarchy of body systems, your lymphatic system would be King. Keeping your lymph system healthy and functioning correctly is of utmost importance before and during a pandemic.

Your blood moves rapidly through your body and makes up only about 1/4th of the fluids in your body. 3/4ths of your fluid is actually your lymphatic fluid. Your lymph fluid is slow moving and is lipid-based which makes it thicker and more mucus-like. It lines your whole body including your lungs, gut, eyes, nose, ears, and mouth. Interestingly, these are the areas in which higher concentrations of the Ebola virus are found.

Your lymphatic system has lymph nodes. These lymph nodes house bacteria which decompose wastes, just like in a septic tank. These bacteria are what keep you healthy and your immune system strong. These are what keep your body clean and functioning properly. It is interesting to note that the Ebola virus is not found concentrated *in* the lymph nodes but only *around* the lymph nodes.

How Stress Impacts Your Lymphatic System

Stress plays a big part in how your lymphatic system functions. This is why it is important not to fear Ebola. *Fear is one of the worst stressors to the body*. When you are stressed, your body dumps cortisol into your blood, which is a stress-fighting hormone. Recent studies have identified a correlation between stress and disease.[30]

Why?

Remember the function of the body's reaction to stress. If you are being chased by a bear, your body is not worried about digesting the food in your stomach or helping you to feel calm and relaxed. Your body wants you far away from the bear so that you can survive! All of the body functions that normally take place in a calm environment are shut down in the face of stress. That way, energy can be directed toward escape and survival. Chemistry that your body generates in a stress-filled environment is very acidic, and your lymph system does not drain well in an acidic environment. In a normal, less-stressful environment, this would only happen on rare occasions (You don't get chased by bears frequently). This is why people often become sick or gets the flu when they are under large amounts of stress. They are becoming auto-intoxicated through dysfunction of the bowels.[31]

There are at least 2 Ebola survivors that attribute their cure to positivity, keeping their mental and emotional stress low, and prayer. In fact, one doctor that had Ebola in Nigeria worked to keep the other patients housed in the isolation ward in good spirits. They found that the death rate in that ward dropped, apparently by this single action.

Your blood, lymph, and your overall body tissues must remain in a very narrow pH range in order for you to stay alive. When your system becomes too acidic, it threatens your survival, and so your body must reduce the acidity quickly. To do that, it takes calcium from the walls of your arteries, veins, bones, and fingernails. However, you need your

---

30 http://www.pnas.org/content/109/16/5995.full

31 http://www.holistichealthtools.com/auto.html

17

calcium in all of those places so that Vitamin D3 (which you will read about a little later) can help keep your body strong.

Getting your lymphatic system working better is not hard to do. Pick and choose what you can work into your life right now and incorporate these on a regular basis if you are ever in the middle of a pandemic outbreak.

Simple Ways to Boost Your Lymphatic System

Here are several easy ways to boost your lymphatic system:

De-stress: Get the stress out of your life. Your life is literally depending on making you and your happiness a priority. Get toxic people out of your life or limit the access they have to you.

Train yourself to relax: The best ways to accomplish this? Learn to meditate, take up yoga, or find some type of practice during which you quiet your mind.

Find happiness: Sometimes this is difficult to do, even in a "normal" world. It can be even harder in the face of scary and challenging times. However, take time now to determine what makes you happy and feel calmer. Then arrange to bring and keep these items and activities in your life should you have to deal with a very stressful situation, whether it be Ebola or something else.

Rest: Make sure you are getting quality sleep. Stay off the electronics at night and turn the TV off. Strive for at least 5 hours of uninterrupted sleep each night in order to get the most benefit.

Food: *"Let food be your medicine, and let medicine be your food." - Hippocrates*

• Focus on quality, not quantity.

• Eat less every day. Consider intermittent fasting as a way to make your cells healthy and strong. You will likely also lose weight, which makes it easier for your immune system to function properly.

• Eat a lot of garlic every day.

• Go raw with 75% of your diet being fresh fruits and vegetables.

Eat for the Season: During the warmer months of Spring and Summer, 80% of your diet should be alkaline. More acidic foods should be incorporated into your diet during the cooler months of fall and winter. You want 60% alkaline foods during these months.

• Eat Beets and drink beet juice.

• Consume a lot of berries and cherries.

• Drink 1 quart of green juice every morning.

• Sip very warm or hot purified water every 10 minutes throughout the day. Add some fresh lemon for even better results. It needs to be hot or very warm water. You need to drink half your weight in ounces with this method. This is the best way to open your cells and really rehydrate your body. *Doing this every day for 2 weeks is a wonderful way to rehydrate each season.* Make sure for the rest of the time that you are staying properly hydrated each day.

Lymph-Moving Therapies:

The following techniques and exercises are focused on keeping your lymphatic fluid moving throughout your body. Find the exercises that feel good to you and practice them regularly to keep your lymph from becoming stagnant.

• Nasal Breathing (also known as a simplified breath of fire): Breathe deeply and rapidly in and out of your nostrils. Your ribs should be noticeably moving in and out. Do this for 2 minutes several times a day. Your ribs are a key mover for your lymphatic system. It helps move toxins out of your intestines and lower body so they can be eliminated. This is an amazing technique to move your lymph:

• Before every shower, massage warmed sesame seed oil (not toasted) or castor oil into your skin. Start from your feet and work your way up your body. Include your face.

• Jumping rope, bouncing gently on a mini-trampoline, or even light jogging are all excellent ways to move your lymph.

• Fruit has a very positive and strengthening effect on your lymphatic system so make sure you consume a lot of fruit in its raw state every day.

Remember, focus on your lymph system and what it takes to get it healthy and keep it healthy. It is directly linked to your immune system and your survival.

Ebola Prep Supplementation (Before Exposure):

The items on the following supplement list have proven to provide benefits that directly address the issues caused by an Ebola virus infection. Read through the list and suggestions and decide which seem right for you. Don't forget to read the footnotes and referenced articles and studies so you'll have confidence in the approach that you are taking.

• **Garlic and fermented black garlic:** Garlic in large doses has been found to have very strong anti-virus activities, especially when taken pre-exposure.[32]

Eat as many cloves of garlic per day as you can. Eating them raw gives you the best protection as cooking destroys some of the medicinal qualities. Cut the garlic cloves open. Pierce many times with a fork and allow to sit on a counter for 15 minutes to activate the properties before eating.

If you are worried about the smell, there are a couple of things you can do. One is to slice the garlic clove in half lengthwise. Then, remove the green sprout-like center from the garlic. Don't eat that part and you will reduce the 'garlic smell' dramatically. The other is to use black fermented garlic.

Black fermented garlic has shown to have almost similar medicinal benefits without the smell or harshness of raw garlic. Black fermented garlic tastes sweet and does not emit an odor. You can easily eat an entire bulb where you could not with regular garlic.

• **Vitamin D3:** Supplementing with D3 is as crucial as is being

---

32 Planta Med. 1992 Oct;58(5):417-23. "In vitro virucidal effects of Allium sativum (garlic) extract and compounds." Weber, Andersen, North, Murray, Lawson, Hughes. Department of Microbiology, Brigham Young University

frequently out in the sun. Vitamin D3 acts as an immune system regulator. It neither stimulates it so much that it causes inflammation and neuro-degeneration nor does it stimulate it too little so that viruses, bacteria and other invaders are left unchecked.[33] Vitamin D also helps protect CD4 T cells, and important part of the body's defense against viruses.[34] Take up to 40,000 IU of a high-quality vitamin D3 daily.

• **Calcium & Vitamin K2:** Both of these need to be taken with Vitamin D3 to get the full benefits of for immune system strengthening and regulation. A low dose of calcium is all you need. I recommend the product Calm. You can find Vitamin K2 in combination with your Vitamin D3.

• **Ginseng and Red Ginseng**. Ginseng can be very powerful or not worth the money you spend on it. It depends on the quality of the ginseng, how and when it was harvested, and the processing method.[35] If you have a good quality ginseng (especially red ginseng) it is powerful for slowing down the depletion of CD4 T-cells.[36] You want to take around 200 to 250 mg per day.

• **Vitamin C:** A message from a doctor that worked with Ebola victims states that "the very first symptoms of Ebola are exactly the same as scurvy," a disease caused by inadequate vitamin C[37]. This doctor states that the level of Vitamin C in a patient's body suffering from Ebola drops to zero. This also explains why the connective tissues easily begin to break down. Vitamin C is imperative to your immune system. People have suspected that the areas most often affected by Ebola are ones where there was severe malnourishment, which means low Vitamin C stores in the tissues.

I recommend you take a few different Vitamin C types: Naturally

---

33 Smolders J, Moen SM, Damoiseaux J, et al. Vitamin D in the healthy and inflamed central nervous system. Journal of Neurological Sciences. 2011 Aug 22.

34 Smolders J, Damoiseaux J. Vitamin D as a T-cell modulator in multiple sclerosis. Vitamins and Hormones. 2011;86:401-28.

35 Jung J-W, Kang H-R, Ji G-E, et al. Therapeutic effects of fermented red ginseng in allergic rhinitis: a randomized, double-blind, placebo-controlled study. Allergy Asthma Immunol Res. April 2011;3(2):103-110.

36Heungsup Sung,1 Sang-Moo Kang,2 Moo-Song Lee,3 Tai Gyu Kim,4 and Young-Keol Cho,. Korean Red Ginseng Slows Depletion of CD4 T Cells in Human Immunodeficiency Virus Type 1-Infected Patients. Clin Diagn Lab Immunol. Apr 2005

37 http://www.jimstonefreelance.com/ebola.html

occurring (in the form of berries like camu-camu and amla), liposomal Vitamin C, and non-GMO ascorbic acid. These should be taken throughout the day.

• Natural Vitamin C in powder form (1 teaspoon AM and PM).

• Liposomal Vitamin C can be taken at 1 packet AM and PM.

• Ascorbic acid should be taken at 3 level teaspoons every 3 hours. This can be taken at the same time as your other Vitamin C in the morning and evening as well.

Selenium: Selenium has shown that it prevented the often deadly mutations in the Avian Flu virus.[38]

It also has shown to increase the power of your T-cells to fight viruses.[39] Selenium deficiency produces fewer and more sluggish lymphocytes. It has also been demonstrated that viruses are less likely to take over a body that has sufficient selenium levels.[40] The duration and intensity of an illness drops with selenium supplementation.

Take 200 mcg daily.

Oreganol Oil P73: The protein shell of the virus breaks down in the presence of Oregano oil and the infectivity of the virus declined after 15 minutes.[41] Oregano oil mixed with water in a spray bottle can also be used as a successful fomite (virus carrying surfaces) sanitizer.

Put 3-5 drops in water or V8 type of juice. It has a strong oregano taste. It can also be applied to skin with a carrier oil like castor oil.

Essential Oils of Clove, Cinnamon and Lemon: Essential oils have an inhibitory effect on influenza virus replication.[42] The protective

---

38 J American College Nutrition 20: 384–88S, 2001; & FASEB Journal 15: 1846–48, 2001; & Journal Nutrition 133: 1463–67S, 2003

39 Nelson HK et al. "Host nutritional selenium status as a driving force for influenza virus mutations." FASEB. 15:1846-8, 2001

40 Taylor, E. W., Ramanathan, C. S.; Theoretical Evidence that the Ebola Virus Zaire Strain May Be Selenium-Dependent: A Factor in Pathogenesis and Viral Outbreaks? The Journal of Orthomolecular Medicine Vol. 10, No.2, 1995;

41 D.H. Gilling, M. Kitajima, J.R. Torrey and K.R. Bright. Antiviral efficacy and mechanisms of action of oregano essential oil and its primary component carvacrol against murine norovirus. Journal of Applied Microbiology. 2014

mechanism found in the outer layer of RNA and DNA viruses breaks down after being exposed to certain essential oils.[43] The exact Mode of Action ("MOA") of essential oils is still not completely understood. However, there is no denying that they are effective.

You can make up a batch of the essential oil blend ahead of time. Use castor oil as a carrier oil and make up a blend that is easy to use. You will need 4 drops of castor oil to each 1 drop of essential oil.

Here is how to put together a useful blend. Do the following:

• 4 drops of castor oil and 1 drop of cinnamon

• 4 drops of castor oil and 1 drop of clove

• 4 drops of castor oil and 1 drop of lemon oil

Repeat through this rotation until you have a good amount prepared together in one glass jar with a tight fitting lid.

For treatment, put 4 drops of the mixture in an empty capsule and take a capsule three times a day. Also use a little of this mixture to rub on the bottom of your feet before bed.

Monolaurin: Monolaurin has great anti-microbial and anti-viral actions. It is essentially a mono-glyceride that interferes with the lipid coated viruses. Here is where this gets exciting. Ebola has a lipid coat that not only protects its own genome and survival, it also helps to gain hold in the human body.[44] Take 3,000 mg daily immediately after knowledge of exposure. Follow with additional doses each day through the entire 21-day incubation period.

Blue Green Algae: This has shown to improve the survival time in mice exposed to the Ebola virus. Blue Green Algae has a protein called

---

42 Garozzo A, Timpanaro R, Stivala A, Bisignano G, Castro A. Activity of Melaleuca alternifolia (tea tree) oil on Influenza virus A/PR/8: study on the mechanism of action. Antiviral Research. 2011 Jan;89(1):83-8. doi: 10.1016/j.antiviral.2010.11.010. Epub 2010 Nov 21.

43 Siddiqui, Y.M., Ettayebi, M., Haddad, A., Al-Ahdak, M.N. Effect of Essential Oils on enveloped viruses: antiviral activity of oregano and clove oils on herpes simplex virus type 1 and Newscastle disease virus. Med Sci Res. 1996.

44 Yuan, J., Zhang, Y., Li, J., Zhang, Y., Wang, L. F., and Shi, Z. (2012). "Serological evidence of ebolavirus infection in bats", China. Virol. J. 9, 236)

CV-N (cyanovirin-N) that works against the virus.[45] It was first discovered to block HIV through sexual transmission by binding to the sugar molecules on its surface and preventing it from getting inside the cells.

Ebola has shown to have similar molecules on its outside envelope and was proven to inhibit Ebola transmission into the cells when tested. The CV-N was given to the mice prior to Ebola infection and then given once a day after infection. Researchers found that survival time was increased. In humans, this extra time could allow the immune system to kill the virus.

There is a lot of controversy over the use of *cyanobacteria* in supplementation so I recommend starting supplementation in the case that Ebola begins to break out in your area. Start with 1 teaspoon in the morning and if exposure occurs, move that to 1 Tablespoon divided up 3x a day.

Research has shown that Spirulina Platensis has shown similar properties as the blue green algae.[46] I recommend the liquid form. Take 1 dropperful 3x a day.

Nanosilver: Colloidal silver has long been a very potent remedy for bacterial infections. The silver binds with the oxygen inside the bacteria and causes the bacteria to die from oxygen starvation. Viruses do not have oxygen carriers. There are some people that are saying that colloidal silver will not slow down Ebola because of this. Wanting to know about nanosilver's effect on viruses, I took to the research papers.

The structure of Ebola actually resembles many other viruses such as HIV and influenza.[47] Ebola has many glycoproteins which both lends

---

45 Barrientos LG, O'Keefe BR, Bray M, Sanchez A, Gronenborn AM, Boyd MR. Cyanovirin-N binds to the viral surface glycoprotein GP1,2 and inhibits infectivity of Ebola virus. Antiviral Res 2003;58:47-56.

46 1) Ayehunie S, et al. Inhibition of HIV-1 replication by an aqueous extract of Spirulina platensis (Arthrospira platensis). J Acquir Immune Defic Syndr Hum Retrovirol 1998;18:7-12; AND 2) Hayashi T, et al. Calcium spirulan, an inhibitor of enveloped virus replication, from a blue-green algae Spirulina platensis. J Nat Prod 1996;59:83-7.

47 Vladimir N. Malashkevich, Brian J. Schneider, Margaret L. McNally, Michael A. Milhollen, James X. Pang, and Peter S. Kim. Core structure of the envelope glycoprotein GP2 from Ebola virus at 1.9-Å resolution. Proc Natl Acad Sci U S A. Mar 16, 1999;

to its virulence but also to its downfall. Each of the glycoproteins has the ability to attach to a cell in your body in many different ways. The glycoproteins also hide the virus from your immune system.

After the glycoprotein has attached to your cell, your cell then cuts off the arm of the glycoprotein, exposing the virus. The virus, configured in a coil, springs out and invades the cell membrane. Here is where nanosilver steps in, by binding to the glycoproteins of the virus and preventing attachment, fusion and infection of the cells.[48]

Because of the potential this holds, I am recommending nanosilver as part of the protocol. *Please note:* this is very different than home generated colloidal silvers. I am completely in support of making silver at home at a fraction of the cost of store-bought brands for treating common illnesses. However, when we are dealing with something like Ebola, nanosilver is what is effective. The medical documentation states that it is the nano-sized[49] particles that are what is effective against viruses.

Colloidal silver (nanosilver) is going to be needed for any post-secondary support in the case that you do contract Ebola and are in the convalescence stage.

I recommend Nutrasilver because that has been the most effective of all silver products I have ever used, including those I made myself. I recommend a dose of 2 droppers full, 3 times per day. You can also put a drop in your eyes and ears. I have even put them in my infant daughter's eyes and regularly use it in my own.

Turpentine: This really is a universal healer. Turpentine has a very long history of being a natural remedy for many health maladies. It has fallen out of favor due to the prevalence and marketing of pharmaceutical drugs. While turpentine may be largely unnoticed and almost ignored in today's world, it has not been forgotten.

Pure gum spirits of turpentine is distilled pine resin, which is used as a

---

48 Liangpeng Ge, Qingtao Li, Meng Wang, Jun Ouyang, Xiaojian Li, and Malcolm MQ Xing. Nanosilver particles in medical applications: synthesis, performance, and toxicity. Int J Nanomedicine. 2014

49 A nanometer (nm) is one billionth of a meter. A nano-sized particle is between 1 nm and 100 nm in size.

natural remedy for many ailments from parasites to soothing joints and muscles to candida. It will kill off microbials, pathogens, viruses, and bacteria.[50] It is also a powerful blood cleanser. These are the reasons I have added it to the Ebola protocol.

Turpentine with which you are probably familiar, used for furniture stripping and cleaning artist's brushes, and commonly found at hardware and paint stores, is mineral turpentine. This is a petroleum distillate and toxic. I do not recommend anyone going to the hardware store to buy turpentine for their body. Pure gum spirits of turpentine is very different.

For a child ages 3-9: Take 1 DROP (with an eyedropper) of pure gum spirits of turpentine with 1 teaspoon of castor oil and with 1 teaspoon of honey. Mix really well for a few minutes and add that to full fat, plain, no sugar yogurt or no sugar, plain coconut yogurt. Take this 2x a week. Follow with a glass of purified water or juice.

For a child age 10-16: Take 4 DROPS (with an eyedropper) of pure gum spirits of turpentine with 1 teaspoon of castor oil and with 1 teaspoon of honey. Mix really well for a few minutes and add that to full fat, plain, no sugar yogurt or no sugar, plain coconut yogurt. Take this 2x a week. Follow with a glass of purified water or juice.

For age 17- Adult: Take 6 DROPS (with an eyedropper) gum spirits of turpentine with 1 Tablespoon of castor oil and mix with 1 teaspoon of honey. Take this before a meal. It can equally be mixed with yogurt and can be taken every other day. Follow with a large glass of purified water.

For adults, this dosage can be increased by 1 DROP (with an eyedropper) gum spirits of turpentine every 7 days until you reach a maximum dosage of 10 DROPS every other day.

You may experience a herxheimer reaction[51] when die-off of occurs.

---

50 Dellanno C, Vega Q, Boesenberg D (2009) The antiviral action of common household disinfectants and antiseptics against murine hepatitis virus, a potential surrogate for SARS coronavirus. Am J Infect Con 37: 649–652.

51 A Herxheimer reaction is an increase in the symptoms of a disease or infection occurring in some persons when

You need to access your health and follow your gut intuition. Herxheimer reactions are normal for many people, but can become overwhelming. If this occurs you should drop your dosage down a bit more until you can handle the die-off and lessen the reaction.

I want to stress that pure gum spirits of turpentine is powerful medicine and not to be abused or taken lightly. ***Do not take more than you should!*** It could cause problems with your liver and kidneys. You need to be healing your body and making it stronger, not weaker. A little bit is a good thing but more than that is abuse.

If Exposed to Ebola (up to the first few days after symptoms begin):

The following additions and dose adjustments are suggested if you should be unlucky enough to be exposed to the Ebola or any other virus.

Vitamin C: You will take only the ascorbic acid form of Vitamin C. You want to take 5,000 mg every 2 hours.

Baking Soda & Apple Cider Vinegar: Dr. Volney Cheney promoted the use of baking soda after understanding its medicinal power during the 1918-1919 deadly virus attacks.[52] He since then used it for viruses, colds and a multitude of other maladies. The apple cider vinegar acts as a synergist.

Use ½ teaspoon of baking soda in 2 Tablespoons Apple Cider Vinegar, taken in 6 ounces of water 3x a day.

Selenium will be increased to 4,000 mcg the first day and 1,000 mcg every day after that.

2% Magnascent iodine: Magnascent iodine is necessary when dealing with viruses, especially lethal influenzas.[53] It is an imperative part of any Ebola treatment.

---

treatment is started, thought to be caused by the massive die-off of the infectious bacteria or virus, and subsequent release of toxins into the body.

52 http://articles.mercola.com/sites/articles/archive/2009/12/15/baking-soda-used-to-treat-swine-flu-85-years-ago.aspx

53 Dr. Donki, J, Chakradhar . Clinical study of efficacy of magnascent iodine (nascent iodine) as therapeutic and chemoprophylaxis agent in tropical malaria. International Scientific Exchange. 2012

• **For Adults (12 years and older):** Take 15 drops in 3.5 ounces of water every 4 hours before food.

• **For Children (5-12 years):** Take 6 drops in 3.5 ounces of water every 4 hours before food.

• **For children under 5:** take 2 drops in 3.5 ounces of water or juice every 4 hours before food.

Bitter Kola Nuts: Garcinia kola (not the much-hyped garcinia cambogia weight loss supplement) has been used as a natural medicine because it is anti-inflammatory, kills parasites, and has proven to be effective against microbes and viruses.[54] It also has very effective liver protective properties, which could be very useful in the case of an Ebola infection. More importantly, Ebola creates an overwhelming amount of free radicals in the body and Kola nuts are powerful free radical scavengers.[55]

While it has been touted as a cure for Ebola, we don't know for sure that it can cure anything. Based on the MOA of bitter Kola, it appears that it slows down the replication of viruses. I added it here simply because places like Instagram are banning people from posting anything about Garcinia Kola.

Simply store the nuts in a jar in pure water in the refrigerator. Eat 1 nut daily. You can also make a nut milk and drink the milk.

Thymus thumps: Your thymus helps to release your killer T-cells. Moderately tap on your thymus which is in the middle of your body, just below your collar bones. It is about where you have seen gorillas beat on their chest. *"Ba-rump, ba-rump, ba-rump, ba-rump."* Do this every 3 hours.

If vomiting or diarrhea makes taking iodine impossible, painting the bottom of the feet with iodine will be the next best choice. Your body

---

54 Farombi, E. O. and Owoeye, O. Antioxidative and Chemopreventive Properties of Vernonia amygdalina and Garcinia biflavonoid. Int J Environ Res Public Health, 2001.

55 Heckel E., Schlagdenhauffen, F., Some African kolas, in their botanical, chemical, and therapeutical aspects. Am Pharm 1884; 56:81-177

will absorb the iodine through your skin. Do this every hour.

Garlic can be smashed and place of the bottom of the feet and wrapped lightly with gauze instead of ingestion. Again, your body will absorb it through your skin.

Essential oils and the Oregano Oil can be rubbed into the bottom of the feet or palms of the hands as well.

Once infected or when symptoms begin:

Should you begin to suffer from vomiting or diarrhea, it is imperative that you drink at least 4.5 to 5 liters of oral fluid therapy plus additional purified water to replace the fluids you are losing.

Here is the recipe to make your own ORS (oral rehydration solution):

• 1 liter of purified water

• 6 level teaspoons of sugar and

• ½ teaspoon of Himalayan salt

• a tiny pinch of **zinc**.

Shake, stir or mix until all ingredients are dissolved. *PLEASE NOTE: These amounts must be exact.* You must drink at least 4.5 liters of the ORS per day.

Dehydration will cause shock, which is one of the main reasons people die from Ebola.

Drink the ORS constantly, no matter what.

When you are having diarrhea, make sure you are drinking at the same time. It may seem like it's going in one end and passing right out to the other end, but keep drinking it.

Keeping as hydrated as possible is a critical step.

I will end this section with a quote from Prof. Akin Osibogun, CMD, LUTH, on how Nigerian doctors defeated Ebola with water:

"The principal thing is the fluid and electrolyte power which will buy the body some time. The body itself is a soldier, fighting the virus, but it is at a disadvantage when it is losing fluid and electrolytes. You also need to encourage the patient, since it was not easy to ask somebody to be drinking, considering there is already fear, panic and so on."

Once infected, you cannot contract Ebola again or have a relapse once you have made it through. You now have some immunity.

In July 2014, a spokesperson for the Colorado Department of Public Health and Environment reported that a man had contracted the pneumonic plague, which is not only rare but very deadly.[56]

So you see, if Ebola turns out to just fizzle away, there is always something else that is a threat to us. We need to protect ourselves when pandemics threaten. It will not always work to put your head in the sand and say, "It won't happen to me" or "It won't happen in MY country."

Times are changing, and plagues & pandemics are evolving. Understand that this strain of Ebola is not the original Zaire virus. This is a mutated form, which is why no one understands fully exactly what is going to happen, or how events might progress.

Don't be an ostrich and don't wait for someone else to do something to take care of the potential problem. Arm yourself with knowledge, and make preparations to take care of yourself and your family in the face of the threat of any pandemic that might come your way, now or in the future.

---

56 http://www.reuters.com/article/2014/07/10/us-usa-colorado-plague-idUSKBN0FF01720140710

SECTION THREE – HOW TO CREATE A SAFE ENVIRONMENT DURING A PANDEMIC

I will tell you, being in Dallas and not sure where Ebola is going next, I have put my family on a quasi-voluntary lock down. We just don't go out in public unless it is needed and the little ones stay home.

I believe that having a choice is really important. I'd much rather voluntarily do something than be forced to do something. I'd rather secure my own family than have the government or military secure them.

I want to keep the control and choices in my own hands. This means I have to prepare. I have the supplements and supplies we need in place and ready. Hopefully, I'll never need them and I am just one of those "weird prepper people". I'm more than willing to be wrong if it means that I am better protected if I am right.

This next part will be how to protect yourself and your family outside of supplementation.

Cleaning

Ebola is part of the envelope virus family. An envelope is a lipid (fat) layer that surrounds and protects the virus. This is also how the virus attaches to your cells. If we break down that fat layer, the virus is rendered ineffective.

You already know that Ebola can live for a certain amount of time on fomite surfaces. A fomite surface can include anything from counters to floors and furniture to clothing and bedding.

I recommend daily sanitizing methods using natural virus killers:

Take a 24 ounce spray bottle filled with purified water, and then add:

• 6 drops of clove oil

• 6 drops of cinnamon oil

• 6 drops of lemon oil, and

• 3 drops of extra strength oregano oil P73

Shake well before each use. Spray surfaces down well.

To launder clothes, I have made my own homemade solution to kill any pathogens, viruses, bacteria or microbes that may attach to fabrics:

• ½ cup of Disodium Phosphate ("TSP")

• 1 cup Borax

Mix together in a glass bowl. Add to this mix:

• 6 drops of clove oil

• 6 drops of cinnamon oil

• 12 drops of lemon oil

• 12 drops of lavender, and

• 3 drops of extra strength oregano oil P73

Mix well until the essential oils are distributed evenly. Add:

• 1 teaspoon of Miracle II Green Soap and mix well until evenly distributed. Then, the mixture must be dried out. I spread my out on a dehydrator sheet and popped it in the dehydrator to remove the moisture.

Alternatively, you can put your oven on the lowest setting. It may not even be a registered temperature on your oven. You want a temperature of about 115 F degrees. Spread your mixture in a thin layer on a cookie sheet and place in the oven, keeping the door ajar until the powder is dry. This could be as little as 15 minutes but may require longer time.

When it is dry, take a large bowl and put the prepared mix that you just dried into the bowl. Add in 2 cups of Borax and 2 cups of washing soda. Mix well until thoroughly blended. Add to an airtight container and use ¼ cup with each load of laundry.

If someone has entered your home that is contaminated:

In the case of infection or suspected infection, your must sanitize your environment as often as possible.

Make sure that you are wearing the proper protective barriers:

• Disposable gloves
• Goggles with a rubber seal around them.
• N95 masks if you only suspect Ebola. Half-face respirators like: 3M, MSA Safety Works, or North Safety masks are needed if someone is infected. The 95 in the N95 means it is only 95% effective, while 5% of particles can come through. N95 are super economical so they are better than nothing in a pinch.
• Plastic bags or protective shoe coverings
• Gowns, Tyvek body suits, or even full body plastic rain suits. You can also buy several of the plastic rain suits and wash them in a disinfecting solution after wearing them.

• Remember gear for little ones. Buying online can offer you more sizing options and better pricing than buying at a medical supply store.

It is recommended to have about a year's worth of protective barrier supplies on hand.

Here are a list of disinfectants that have shown to be effective at killing Ebola as well as many other pandemic viruses and bacteria.

Envelope Virus Disinfectants:

SOLUTION ONE - Accelerated Hydrogen Peroxide Surface Disinfectant. Here are a few brands that are effective:

- 7% Virox
- PerCept Concentrate
- Accel Surface Cleaner Disinfectant Concentrate

SOLUTION TWO - .05% Accelerated Hydrogen Peroxide Tuberculocidal Surface Disinfectant. Hare are effective brands to consider:

- Oxivir Tb RTU
- Carpe Diem Tb RTU
- Accel TB RTU

All of the brands listed above also come in wipes which make cleaning easier.

SpectraSan Ygiene 206 - Dilution for this will is 2 ounces of disinfectant to 32 ounces of water. To make a gallon, add 9 ounces of liquid to 1 gallon of water.

Clorox Commercial Solutions:

- Hydrogen Peroxide Disinfecting Wipes and Liquids

- Clorox Germicidal Bleach

It is important to note that Clorox has not received certification for their products being able to kill Ebola. The following was posted on their website:[57]

"Currently, the Ebola virus is not available for efficacy testing in the United States. There are no surface disinfectant products with an EPA- registered claim to kill the

---

[57]http://www.cloroxprofessional.com/assets/Industry/Cleaning/Ebola-and-EV68/NI-26965-Ebola-HF-Pathogen-Education.pdf

Ebola virus. However, the CDC recommends the use of EPA registered hospital disinfectants with label claims for non-enveloped viruses to disinfect environmental surfaces in hospitals housing patients with known or suspected Ebola virus infection".

Alternatives:

The CDC suggests the following as an alternative sanitizing solution.[58] Regular household use (unscented) Clorox (5-6% bleach): 1 cup bleach per 5 gallons of water.

The last thing you want to do is use aerosol sprays like Ozone in a can or Lysol type of sprays. The disturbance caused by the spray from an aerosol spray could cause contaminated dust particles to become airborne.

The Decontamination "Safe House" Procedure:

Once you are properly dressed in protective gear, wipe down all surfaces, including furniture, door handles and light switches. Change the wiping cloth when dirty. Dispose of cloths in a large plastic container with a lid that has been properly marked as a biohazard.

Allow surfaces to dry for at least 5 minutes. All fabric must be washed, including curtains. Place into heavy duty garbage bags for laundering.

When leaving a room and before entering another one, wipe your gear and protection down with the Clorox and water solution mentioned above. Wait 3-5 minutes, then take off your protective gear in the doorway and discard into garbage bags that are marked for disposal or washing. To prevent exposure and infection, be careful not to allow your protective gear to touch any part of you as you are taking it off.

Wash hands well and put on new gloves.

For more information, google the following references:

APIC, Ready Reference to Microbes, 2002

Infection Control Guidelines: Hand Washing, Cleaning, Disinfection and Sterilization in Health Care, Health Canada. Dec 1998, Vol 24S8

---

58 http://www.bt.cdc.gov/disasters/bleach.asp

Routine Practices and Additional Precautions for Preventing the Transmission of Infection in Health Care, Health Canada. July 1999, Vol 25S4

Guidelines for Environmental Infection Control in Healthcare Facilities, CDC.

MMWR June 2003, Vol 52, No RR-10 Best Practices for Cleaning, Disinfection and Sterilization in All Health Care Settings, PIDAC, May 2006

Rutala WA & Weber DJ. The benefits of surface disinfection. AJIC 2004;32(4) 226-229

Additional Measures

It is also recommended to fog a room with a solution of 5-6% hydrogen peroxide. You can also run an ozone generator in the room. These will kill the viruses in areas that you may not have been able to reach.

Laundering Suspected Ebola Infected Materials

Most of the above solutions can be added to the laundry. It is imperative that you soak fabrics in one of the above solutions for 30 minutes before laundering. Remember, Clorox will bleach out any fabrics so you may want to use one of the other suggested disinfectants.

Now that you know how to keep your home sanitized, let's move on to prepping in the event that you or a loved one is infected or the area that you are in becomes under Martial Law.

Feeding Your Family

I am fasting type of person. I fast for short and long periods. I have come to realize that when it comes to fasting, I'm standing in the corner by myself. Not many people want to join me. I've fasted for many reasons. I wanted to prepare my body and spirit in case there wasn't the food I was used to. I wanted to detox some age old poisons out to allow for more vibrant health. Fasting helped me to break food addictions. I've also fasted for spiritual reasons. Purifying my mind has been one of the greatest decisions I have made for myself.

I advocate fasting. It's healthy for people to understand they won't go into convulsions and die because they do not get 3 meals a day. I suggest people begin with intermittent fasting. Dedicate a certain amount of hours every day that you will go without food. It slowly trains the body to adapt to the unknown. It also creates great strength in your cells. Cellular strength and integrity is needed in today's world.

Next: unless you are growing your own food, it will be difficult to have fresh food in the event of martial law or any type of lockdown. There are several things you can do. You can dehydrate food. Dehydrated food takes up very little room and lasts for a very long time.

Purchase food that is filling and is easy to store, has a long shelf life and is easy to make. Rice fits into this category. You don't even need electricity to eat rice; you can soak it in water and sprout it to eat it. This goes for quinoa and whole grains. Oatmeal is another food with loads of nutrition that can be stored for a long period of time and still provide sustenance.

It is recommended to have enough food and supplies to last for at least a 90-day period. Six months to a year's worth is even better. However, not everyone is in a position to do this. Just start wherever you are at and don't be discouraged if you cannot buy it all at once. Buy what you can, when you can.

It doesn't matter if you never need your stock because of a pandemic event. You can (and should) rotate your supplies into your regular meal plans. Use a part of your supplies in your day-to-day life, and replace those items as soon as possible. Most people feel more secure when there is access to plenty of food or when the refrigerator and pantry is fully stocked. This takes a HUGE amount of stress and fear away that often happens in pandemic or other lockdown-type situations.

There are three ways that you can prepare to feed yourself and your loved ones during an Ebola outbreak. You can use gardens, both indoor and outdoor and you can begin to store food right now for your survival.

Easy and Unique Food Storage Ideas
Many people went and stockpiled food for Y2K and look how that

turned out. Last time I checked, my computer was still booting up OK. I still see people selling their stock on craigslist now that the food is getting close to expiring.

Adding a few food necessities with each paycheck will help you get closer to your goals step-by-step instead of trying to buy everything at once. Starting now will also protect you in case there is a food shortage. That happened when some of the towns were quarantined in Africa. It has also happened here when the threat of hurricanes came.

You already know that fresh food has a short shelf-life. I already mentioned dehydrating fruits and vegetables because, once dehydrated, they take up a small amount of space and taste great.

If food is kept cool and dry, many times it will exceed its expiration date. If it smells bad or looks molded, rotted or full of bugs, you may want to pass on eating it. In that case, work it into the soil of your garden and let the soil bacteria break it down for you. Extreme temperatures and moisture often will ruin food even before the expiration date.

Beans: You already know that beans are a magical fruit ("the more you eat, the more you…" - oh never mind), but they also make good high-nutrition food for long-term storage. I've already mentioned rice and whole grains.

Powdered Milks & Powdered Coconut Milk: Powdered milk and powdered coconut milk can be very important for you. These can last for years and even decades. There are natural and organic baby formulas that taste pretty good and can supply you with nutritional needs. Because they are packed in cans and are dry powders, the will last quite a while and maintain their nutrition.

Nuts and Nut Butters: Peanut butter and other nut butters are great to keep around. Sunflower seeds and pumpkin seeds are great to snack on, especially for kids. Brazil nuts are a great source of selenium. Make sure the nuts are vacuum-packed and they will remain fresh and provide a source to fulfill important nutrition needs.

Healthy Oils: Consider oils like coconut and olive oil. Coconut oil is not only extremely healthy for you (it's loaded with medium chain triglycerides), it can be eaten cooked or uncooked as well as being applied to hair and skin. Olive oil has many health benefits and will store for a long time in sealed bottles or gallon cans. Stock up on both of these powerhouses.

Rice Crackers: When my kids have peanut butter and jelly, they will have it on very thin non-GMO rice crackers. Rice crackers will keep for a long time if kept away from moisture, and these are much healthier than bread made from bleached out wheat flour. Seal them in a vacuum-packed pouch and they will stay fresh for months.

Sweeteners: Keep a good stock of raw honey because of the enzymes and nutrition. Honey will store indefinitely and retain all of its nutrition. Raw honey and turmeric powder can also be applied to wounds to keep them from getting infected.

Coffee and Tea: Instant coffee and tea is good for variety, stores easily, and is easy to make.

EmergenC: This brand of vitamin C makes a fizzy, vitamin-packed and good-tasting drink in just seconds. Packets of EmergenC are great to stock up on. Kids love the taste of EmergenC as well.

Canned foods: These can be purchased cheaply and put away for a rainy day. If nothing comes of the Ebola pandemic, you can always donate them at Christmas time to the canned food drives, or work them into your family meal plans.

Salt & Spices: Seriously consider stocking up on spices and non-iodized salt. These will greatly help the taste of food, add variety and give you valuable nutrients. I dehydrate a lot of garlic and just grind it into a powder when I want to use it. Cayenne and turmeric, along with Italian spices are popular to store. But, by all means, stock up on salt. In my opinion, it's better to use natural varieties like Himalayan or Celtic Sea Salt. Decide what kind makes sense for you and put some back, along with spices that will add variety to your diet in a lockdown scenario.

Comfort Foods: For many people, a day without chocolate is not a good day. Knowing this, it's a good idea to include comfort foods like chocolate and other long shelf-life treats that will provide welcome happiness (along with the release of "feel-good" endorphins) during a lock-down, quarantine situation.

Good Starter Foods

The foods you want to start with in stocking up are foods like flour, peanut butter, sugar, seeds, honey, tea, lard, oils, coffee and canned goods. While some people don't necessarily think of canned goods as staples, when it comes to surviving, they are.

Water and Water Storage Ideas

Don't forget about water! While collecting rain water is now illegal in a lot of states, if you have some privacy, you can still do it. Also, look into water purification and collection techniques. NOTE: There is more about the importance of water in the next section.

You may consider bottled water. A garage and even a garage attic are both great places in which to store water.

You should double bag food or purchase special food containers to keep out the bugs and critters. I would still place the food in plastic storage totes whether it is in specialty containers or not. These plastic totes can often be found for under $10 at large retail stores like Wal-Mart or Target.

Try to get as much of the air out of your food when you store it in bags as possible. Vacuum-packing is best.

Don't focus on purchasing freezer food because power is not always reliable. If you have ever lost a well-stocked freezer full of food due to a power outage you know how irritating this can be. Concentrate on foods with a long shelf-life that can be stored at room temperature.

Figure out what you would like your staples to be and begin today.

Other Non-Food Essentials

You want your necessities met so you will not have to leave your home to go to the store. What are things you need now that are necessities? These are many of the same items you will need to keep in stock during a pandemic outbreak.

- Toilet paper
- Heavy-duty garbage bags that will not rip easily.
- Shampoo and hair products
- Soap
- Toothbrushes, toothpaste, floss and the original amber colored Listerine.
- Dish soap
- Laundry soap
- Clorox
- Clorox wipes
- Paper towels
- Plastic drop cloths
- Toys
- Games
- Batteries
- Books
- Candles
- Lighters
- Pet food
- Diapers if you have a smaller child
- Adult diapers (needed in case of infection)
- Batteries
- First aid supplies
- Band-Aids
- Tampons or sanitary napkins
- Hibiclens disinfectant soap
- Calamine Lotion
- 100 proof vodka
- A couple of buckets
- Mason Jars
- Plastic totes and tubs
- Large outdoor garbage cans
- 1 gallon glass jugs
- Utilities knives
- A few Leatherman's multi-tool pliers and/or Swiss Army knives
- Thermal blankets.
- Thermometers (non battery-powdered)
- Solar powered radio
- Walkie-talkies or 2-way radios.

• Extra sets of blankets, clothes, socks, underwear, shoes, and coats for everyone in the family. Seal these, and keep them away from the house if possible.
• Herbal and OTC medicines for non-Ebola related issues like: headaches, stomach aches, indigestion, sore throats, fevers, diarrhea, vomiting, allergic reactions, and chest colds.
• Prescription medicines that have to be taken. Most doctors will give you a 6 month to 1 year supply of a prescription if you ask for it and tell them you are ordering from an online pharmacy.
• More chocolate…

Start an Indoor Garden

Not only does growing food bring you satisfaction, but it provides you a way to eat abundantly without having to go to the store.

Berries are some of the best food for keeping your immune system strong. Fruit is very filling; much more filling than vegetables.

Blueberries can be grown indoors. There are compact varieties. Blueberries generally do not produce fruit the first year, so get started now.

Strawberries are another fruit that can be grown with ease inside. When you get the varieties that are long producers, you can have extended seasons of growing.

Tomatoes, greens and kale can all be grown indoors. Cherry tomatoes are proliferate producers. Greens can be cut down to 2" from the stem and will regrow 3-4 times.

A garden will not help you in the next month, but it will be a huge asset in the future. Seeds are still available at many health food markets and online so get started.

The end of a growing season is a great time to pick up planting and gardening supplies for inexpensively at your local stores. If not, there are also Amazon and other online sellers.

Lighting may be a concern for many people. Plants need light to grow. There are lights that can mimic the sun that will help you grow your food indoors or out.

There are basic grow bulbs to more expensive metal halide lamps. Choose what is best and most affordable for your needs.

Consider Hidden Gardens

People do weird and unpredictable things when faced with a fearful situation. Look at the looting that has gone on in the past. It is a good idea not to broadcast that you are becoming self-sustainable because you never know how people will react in a time of desperation.

Even if you have a large family and not a lot of space for gardening, there are some easy ways to grow your own food.

Container gardening and vertical gardens are great ways to maximize small spaces. Most people only know the appearance of basic food. Planting lesser known varieties of vegetables, herbs and fruits allow for you to hide edibles in your flower gardening and landscaping.

People rarely think food can be potted in planters. For example: sweet potato vines are used as ornamental landscaping plants for their bright yellowy green leaves, but underneath the plants is real food. Many plants look ornamental but are actually food. Check out Markus Rothkranz's Edible Plant guide.

If you have a lot of land, consider just throwing a bunch of seeds out and letting whatever germinates together to grow. To the average person this will probably look like a messy, unkempt yard, but to you this is a lot of food with little to no care taking.

If there is an empty lot or unused land near your house, you may consider throwing some seeds in there to grow food. People will never think to go foraging in a vacant lot, but you will have plenty of food for you and your family. It will be sort of a set it and forget it type of gardening.

If it is far enough away from the road, it will blend in with the surroundings, which is what you want.

Voluntary Quarantine

Voluntary quarantines can keep you and your family safe. If you do a semi-quarantine, this gives your family good practice and helps you to know what to modify to fit your family's needs.

Outside of vacations, it's the one time that you can spend just being with the people you love the most during an extended period of time. If you don't like the people you would spend time with, then maybe reconsider who is around you. Getting along, having harmony and happiness will go over much better than arguing, bickering and anger. You need to feel safe with the people that surround you. You have to know that everyone is working for others and not just for the safety, security and comfort of themselves.

This is the hardest part. In stressful situations, most people will operate on automatic and instinct. If someone's instinct is to secure their comfort over another or to operate like they are a single being without regard for the others around them that bears some deep thought.

Stress usually brings out to the worst in people. You need to know how to mitigate as much stress as possible, and this skill is developed with practice. Ebola is not being announced as all over Dallas at this time, but I am using this stretch to practice as much as possible. It also is a change for us to not get up and just go out for the sake of just getting out of the house.

Why would you want to practice voluntary quarantine procedures?

If you've heard any news outlet talking about Ebola, you will hear the terms isolation and quarantine once someone is infected. As much as we may not like that, that is actually one of the best ways to stop the spread of any pandemic situation.

You already know that people are only mildly contagious before they are showing full blown Ebola symptoms, but your focus should always be on how to keep others safe and stop the spread of the virus.

The experience of the Firestone compound located in Harbel, Liberia is a great example of how to contain and stop the spreading of Ebola.

What they instituted there has saved the lives of countless people.[59] We can do the same thing here in our own homes.

When a pandemic breaks out in your area, it is much wiser to go into a voluntary quarantine instead of going about your normal routine of visiting people, shopping, eating out and seeking outside entertainment.

My spouse gave me a $20 bill last night and asked me if money is a fomite. The answer is yes. So are seats in a movie theater or chairs and linens at a restaurant. Speaking of restaurants, how many times have you sat down to dinner and noticed lipstick still on a glass, or dirty utensils? I can guarantee you that most restaurants do not have the proper sanitation in place to completely kill a pandemic virus.

If Ebola shows up in your area, it is not worth it to try to pretend it is not around. The more people around you, the faster the virus will be spreading. There will always be the majority of people unprepared and in denial. You cannot rely on other people to protect you and your family, you have to do it.

Let's say Ebola breaks out full force in your town and people are forced to realize the gravity of the situation, what is the first thing they are going to do? Panic! People will try to leave the area, which will only result in a forced military quarantine. This is NOT a situation you want.

You have a couple of options. You can leave to a pre-determined destination before people catch on to how big this really is, or you can hunker down in your own home. The fact is that you can't tell who is contagious or who is safe.

People can start to show symptoms from a few days to three weeks before people show the clinical symptoms of Ebola. It took Thomas Duncan a week and he was here in Dallas the majority of that time. You don't want to rely on killing the virus after you have it; you want to avoid getting it in the first place. This is where preparation comes into place.

59http://www.npr.org/blogs/goatsandsoda/2014/10/06/354054915/firestone-did-what-governments-have-not-stopped-ebola-in-its-tracks

I suggest having a place to go outside of your area. This puts the control totally back into your own hands. If you stay, you are never sure what will happen. There may be forced vaccinations, you could be separated from your family against your will, or there could be government mandated blood draws from all of your family members. I can tell you that in a scenario like that, it is unlikely you'll be treated with kindness and respect. You will be treated as a number, not a person. No one likes that especially in a scary situation. The military has been prepped for this for a long time. You do not want to be a statistic if you can help it.

Plan ahead with a meeting point where everyone can meet up. Make sure someone is in charge of bringing your prep gear ready, since you should already have this packed and ready to go just in case.

If you can't avoid going out, avoid crowds. If you've taken my advice, you will already have your necessities stocked and will not really have a need to go out. If you find that you have to go out, wear a face mask to prevent inhaling the virus. Only touch surfaces you absolutely have to and wear protective gloves. Yes, you will look like a freak, but you will be a smart freak.

You will have to take a very firm stance on protecting yourself and your family. You cannot allow people in or out; even a neighbor. On that note, do not answer the door if people come to it. Remember, most people will have not prepared and most people are selfish by nature. Not out of meanness, just out of a lifetime of doing what is best for them and not looking at the ripple effect of their actions.

Do not give your power over to someone else. Do not put your life in the hands of someone else. People will drop the ball; it has become human nature. It doesn't matter what you want the reality to be, it only matters what the true reality actually is.

Steps to Quarantine an Exposed or Infected Person
You have to think like a doctor. This is where watching all those doctor shows on television might actually come in handy. Research what is happening to people when they are suspected of having Ebola. People are immediately put into quarantine.

There is not a lot of contact with that person and very specific protocols are put into place as precaution. This prevents the spread. This is why you need plans put into place ahead of time. You need to know how to take care of a loved one and how to protect everyone else in your home. Remember, it doesn't matter if they look sick or feel sick.

A quarantine room cannot be in your house. It can be in the garage, as long as your supplies are not kept there. The best is to have a tent outside. I caution a garage if it is attached to your house. A tent is best.

I suggest investing in a heavy duty tent that can house as many people as you have in your family. The heavy duty tents will help protect against weather changes. Make sure that any mesh on your tent can be completely secured. Remember, Ebola can travel on droplets and can be airborne in that sense. You want to completely contain the virus. The cabin style tents usually have windows and doors that can be completely zipped up. Many often have areas where you can run electricity into the tent in a secure manner.

Set up the tent far enough from your house that you will not risk other people but close enough that you can be alerted if they should need help. Walkie-talkies and cell phones are great to have on hand. Cell phones or computers that allow you to see the person will be very valuable. You may also want to consider having a baby video monitor in the case that someone is too ill to work a computer. This will allow you to see what is going on inside the tent. Someone should be in isolation for the full 3 weeks or for 1 week after the symptoms stop.

As hard as this is, the person that is quarantined will have to remain alone as much as possible. This will be very hard but will have to be abided by for the best protection. Do not enter the isolation tent unless you absolutely have to.

When it comes to isolating kids, this is especially emotionally difficult as they may not understand. Have plenty of toys, books, games and electronics to keep them busy. Know that whatever is in the isolation tent will have to be disposed of and cannot be taken out with the person once they are well.

Preventative Steps to Avoid Non-Ebola Ailments (aka the flu)

Think about how quickly a cold or the flu goes around, tearing through schools and offices. You also have to prepare for non-Ebola illnesses. When you are in a stressful situation, your immune system will always be compromised so it is important to do what you can to prevent illness instead of treating it once it hits.

Vitamin C is an important part of your arsenal. There are debates between buffered and non-buffered, but the fact is, they all work. Get whatever one you agree with. Try to purchase non-GMO forms. You will want to take between 2,000-4,000 mg per day.

Be aware of something called "bowel tolerance" when you are taking preventative doses of vitamin C. Everyone has a different level at which they will begin to have diarrhea when taking large doses of vitamin C orally. Start with 500 mg per day and work your way up to the recommended dose by increasing your dosage by 500 mg per day.

When you begin to 'loosen up' then back off to the previous level. This will be your maintenance dose for prevention. If you should start to feel ill, move back up until you reach bowel tolerance again. Likely, your maintenance dose will be higher when fighting off a bug like a cold or the flu.

You will want to save your specific Ebola supplements discussed earlier in the event that Ebola strikes you or your family. You will be stocking up in bulk.

Take your Multivitamins. While under normal circumstances I do not recommend a multi-vitamin and mineral supplement, in the case of an Ebola outbreak I suggest you have some bulk multi-vitamin and mineral supplements on hand, especially if you end up in a quarantine situation (voluntary or otherwise).

Normally you should be getting your nutrition from your food. In a non-quarantine situation, you are free to make healthy food choices but in a dire circumstance you probably will not have that luxury. When this is the case, it is better to use an all-in-one supplement than to do without.

Get a separate B-vitamin complex. This will keep you calm and your brain healthy. Vitamin B is needed for your neuro-health. It will help to keep you calm cool and collected.

Stock up on vitamin D3. D3 is hugely important to your immune system.

Rescue Remedy. Rescue Remedy is great for kids, adult and animals. It really takes the edge off of stress effectively. Have some in your medicine cabinet.

Zinc. Zinc is another powerhouse that keeps your body strong, even under stress.

Apple Cider Vinegar and Aluminum Free Baking soda. At the first sign of a cold, taking ¼ teaspoon baking soda and 2 Tablespoons of apple cider vinegar in 6 ounces of water will knock and cold or flu out flat. Make sure you mix it well before taking. Take this 3x a day until you are symptom free. If you are in full blown symptoms, take ½-1 teaspoon of baking soda and 2 Tablespoons of apple cider vinegar in 6 ounces of water. Take this 3x a day until you are symptom free.

Yin Chiao Formula: If taken at the first sign of a cold, it will knock it out. This Chinese herbal remedy is good for fever, sore throat, nasal congestion, upper respiratory viruses, chicken pox, and measles. Good to take for viruses. Take 1 pill 4x a day.

Huang Lien Formula: Antibacterial. Good for high fevers, strep throat, sinus and eye infections, ear infections, sties, tonsillitis, and headaches. Good to take for bacterial infections. Take 1 pill 4x a day.

Nin Jiom Pei Pa Koa Syrup by Dragon Herbs. This is amazing for sore throats and to clear a cough really quick. Good for children as well and it's good tasting.

All 3 of these herbal formulas are very inexpensive and can be found online or at your local Asian market.

I'd love to say that quality matters and if you are in the situation to stock up on a lot of quality supplements, do that. If you are on a limited budget go to your local big box store like Walmart and find the supplements that can offer you the highest values. If you can find Vitamin D3 in 10,000 IU, get that versus a 1,000 IU dose.

Just buy them in bulk. Bulk warehouses like Sam's Club and Costco are great ways to save money and buy in large quantities. Do not worry about expiration dates. Rarely do expiration dates hold any real meaning, especially if the items are stored properly and have not been subject to wide swings in temperature.

Turmeric is truly a wonder spice. It can be mixed with honey and applied to wounds to prevent infection or taken in high doses to prevent you from getting sick. There is no known level of toxicity with turmeric with extensive research data showing its safety and efficacy.

Black garlic. I am going to continue to sing the praises of black garlic. While it is more expensive than regular garlic, it can be taken in high doses and has potent properties that can keep you healthy. Because it is already fermented, it will not go bad and the taste is pleasant enough for kids. It has shown to be effective against the influenza virus.

Colloidal Silver (NutraSilver) will prevent pink eye with the first signs of red eyes and itchiness. You can also keep home brewed colloidal silver on hand. Please remember that home brewed colloidal silver is not strong enough for Ebola but works wonders for a lot of other maladies.

Activated Charcoal. This is cheap and the best remedy for food poisoning, diarrhea and upset stomach. Take 6 capsules every hour until affliction passes.

For the more adventurous and daring, keep an enema bucket and a purging tea like Smooth Move. Part of keeping yourself healthy is your ability to remove waste from your body at least once a day, but preferably several times a day.

More About Water
Did you know that a healthy immune system is directly correlated to

water intake? Because your immune system is regulated by your lymphatic system, a lymph system won't move if the lymph fluid is thick and sluggish. Drinking plenty of water will help your lymph system move easier which will enhance your immunity!

Most people are mildly dehydrated and they are not even aware of it. Many research papers and books have been written about the effects of mild dehydration on the body. It is amazing how quickly symptoms clear once the body is properly rehydrated over time.

For instance, if you are having an asthma attack, did you know that drinking a cup of strong coffee and then following that with drinking about a liter of water with a pinch of salt in it will slow down and often stop and asthma attack altogether? This works on children as well. The water will have to be adjusted according to the size and age of the child, but it works. Drinking a quart of water with a pinch of salt is a preventative measure against having an asthma attack. Both of these anti-asthma remedies work; I have had many firsthand experiences with these in children and adults.

I've already shown to you the importance of hydration when you have Ebola to prevent shock and slowing down your lymph system, so why not hydrate your body on a regular basis. We do not know if this single action could prevent you from ever getting Ebola in the first place. Regardless, the health benefits are worth it.

Long-Term Storage of Water
If you figure that each adult should have between 3-4 liters of water a day, you will have a rough idea of how much water to have on hand. It's important not to forget about your pet's need for water too.

Opaque, food-grade 55 gallon plastic drums can often be found on Craigslist for around $20 to $35 (at the time of writing of this book, anyway). Tuck several of these in a corner of your garage, fill them with water, and then prepare the water for long-term storage by adding a little iodine and/or a bit of bleach using the formulas below. You'll have a source of water for consumption during a long quarantine should tap water become unavailable.

NOTE: If you're going the 55 gallon drum route, be sure to place the drums where you want them BEFORE you fill them up. Water weighs about 8 pounds per gallon, so your 55 gallon drum is going to top out at around 440 pounds! Also, make sure you can access the drums where they will be stored. The water can be removed with a hose by siphoning it out.

For a 55 gallon drum, add 2 ounces of 2% iodine before sealing the drum. NOTE: Some people are allergic to iodine. One sign that there may be an iodine allergy is if there is an allergy to shellfish. In that case, you can use bleach to prepare the water for long-term storage.

For a 55 gallon drum, add 7 teaspoons (or 1 ounce plus 1 teaspoon) of common household bleach (5% to 6%) before sealing the drum. Be sure to use freshly purchased bleach.

At minimum, you should have 1 weeks' worth of water for each person stocked up.

In the case that water to your house should be compromised, make sure you have extra water set aside for hygiene, cleaning, and washing.

There should also be an additional water stash put aside for each person in the case that the oral rehydration solution is needed.

You can also use smaller containers. Many juices come in 1 gallon glass bottles. Drink the juice, clean the bottles, and re-fill with water. Store your water containers wrapped in opaque black plastic bags keeps it safe and protected. A dark closet is also a good storage location. To prolong the shelf life of stored water, group the gallons or bottles in opaque containers and place those containers in dark plastic bags. This keeps the light out and keeps the water fresher for longer periods of time.

You can buy cheap 2.5 gallon jugs or stock 5 gallon bottles and have a dolphin hand pump to get the water out with ease. Just be sure to use food grade containers for long-term storage. Avoid water that has fluoride in it, if possible. Distilled is best.

To store large quantities, like the 55 gallon drums discussed earlier, you can use tap water, and then filter the water before consumption. Filters like the Adya multi-stage filter or a Berkey water filter will help clean up the water before consumption.

Do not store your water near chemicals or other hazardous materials. Keep your water safe because this is the most vital part of your survival.

Make sure you keep your water supply stored away from chemicals or odorous things like gasoline, bleach, and pesticides. Water can absorb other odors. You should check your water supply every few months to ensure the gallons or bottles are still sealed tightly and that none of the containers have started leaking.

It is equally important to know if you have a fresh water supply close to you should the public water supply fail. You can also buy food safe barrels to collect water in. All you will have to do in both of these cases is purify the water.

Water Purification Methods

You could potentially find yourself in a situation where your water supply is suspect, even if it coming through the pipes in your home. One study suggests that it would only take around 10% of the workforce being off the job to dramatically disrupt the delivery of utilities, including water and electricity.

You can buy chlorine purification tablets online or at any camping or outdoor type store. Buy these in bulk for easy purification. They will easily stay good for a couple of years. You can also buy powdered chlorine used to shock pools, calcium hypochlorite. The powdered chlorine has an indefinite shelf-life, while liquid household bleach only maintains the 5% to 6% concentration for about 6 months, up to 12 months at best according to the Clorox Company. A small, one pound container will treat up to ten thousand gallons of water. Plus, it can be used as a disinfectant for surfaces as well. It comes in a range of different levels of purity (usually between 68% to 73%), so be sure to get at least 68% purity.

Here is a fairly simple formula: Add 1 teaspoon of powdered pool shock to one gallon of water.[60] An old gallon bleach bottle works well for this. Then, dilute this mixture 1 to 100 in order to purify water. So, for example, if you want to purify a five-gallon jar, the math is as follows:

1 gallon = 128 ounces, so 5 gallons = 640 ounces

Divide 640 ounces by 100, and you get 6.4 ounces

Add 6.4 ounces (go ahead and round up to 6 ½ ounces) to the five gallon container, and let it sit for at least 30 minutes.

Don't skimp on purifying your water, because you could get very sick. Most of the lake and river water supplies are greatly contaminated, with Giardia and Cryptosporidium are found within the USA. These will make you horrifically sick and can be fatal.

A quick and effective way to purify water without all the calculations and measuring and pouring is through the use of purification tablets. These tablets can be bought at camping stores or through online stores. One tablet only purifies one liter of water, so you'll need to have a bulk supply of these.

Always strain your collected rainwater twice by placing a towel or even a coffee filter over the top of a bowl. Pour your collected water through that into your container. Repeat.

If you have the means to boil the water, I suggest boiling it for 10 minutes. This will absolutely assure the elimination of harmful parasites. Add bleach solution according to the formulas already discussed above. Shake the bottle to mix the water inside and allow it to sit for a few hours with only a paper towel over the top.

Add a few drops of Magnascent iodine to your water, seal your bottles well and shake.

Magnascent iodine is needed because there are some microscopic parasites that are immune to chlorine. Using the last step with

---

60 http://www.backdoorsurvival.com/how-to-use-pool-shock-to-purify-water/

Magnascent iodine will kill everything in your water. (NOTE: Do not use iodine for water purification if anyone in your household is allergic to iodine, or be sure to filter the water thoroughly before consumption).

If purified properly and stored correctly, your bottled water will be fine in storage for a couple of years. Make sure you write a date on your water so you know when it was purified and stored.

Other Potential Pandemics

The point of this book is not just to give you a fighting chance against Ebola; it's to give you a fighting chance against any pandemic that might land on your doorstep.

Ebola is scary and there is a lot of fear being spread around about it. The reality is that any dangerous pandemic can be a scary situation. Remember how scared people were of the Bird Flu, SARS or MRSA (the 'flesh-eating' virus)?

There are other plagues and pandemics that are in every state across America right now in one form or another. They are killing people are we just are not hearing about it in main stream media, especially with the spot light on Ebola.

You probably have not heard about H5N1 which is one of the deadliest avian flu viruses yet or the H7N9 which some researchers fear will become a horrible pandemic. Until recently, both of these had only been found in avian (bird) populations, but have since mutated and jumped to human hosts.

Researchers are warning that it is just as matter of time before one or more of these viruses mutate enough to spread to pandemic proportions. We are seeing a big trend in animal viruses that are infecting humans. Like Ebola, we are uncertain to just how bad this could get.

Closer to home, it is the yearly flu that is posing the most looming danger to us because we have come to accept its norm in our lives. We don't think it's a big deal when someone has the flu, yet it has been mutating out of control and each year becomes stronger, more resistant and kills more elderly, men, women and children. If you think your flu shot is protecting you, you are wrong. Last year's flu strain is what is in your vaccine. That flu virus has mutated so much; your vaccine does not protect you from the new strain.

There are no credible research papers that show that last year's strain of flu virus prevents this year's flu. It is all propaganda. Why? I don't know. People continue to stand by their vaccine because they feel helpless. They've failed to educate themselves on their own body and how to stay healthy so they don't feel they can change their minds; there's too much insecurity in that. Most people know that they are not truly healthy anyway. They have no many aches, pains and afflictions. But like the society we are, we turn a blind eye to the truth and ask for warm and fuzzy illusions instead.

These animal spread and lab created viruses have the real potential to strike and kill families, communities and devastate countries. We are not like Africa were people are living very spread out and something can be isolated or ignored with ease. There is very little open land left in America and that puts any pandemic that strikes into something that should be considered a very serious situation. People in California will not be disconnected from the ravages that Texas may see from Ebola. It will only be a matter of weeks after a spread that it hits there too.

I am saddened by the people that choose to believe that Ebola is a hoax and ignore preparation of any kind. You see, it's just not Ebola that we are working against. I wish more people understood that. Preparation, 'prepping,' or whatever you want to call it brings peace of mind in case something happens. If there is not a pandemic that strikes, what did your prepping hurt?

I don't believe it's a good idea to walk around and tell people about prepping. The majority of people just will not understand and will either ridicule you or attack you. It's a strange position to be in. You will be accused of spreading fear instead of what you are actually doing, which is helping to increase prevention and personal responsibility.

People that are unprepared and caught off-guard are the ones that are more likely to panic and create a worse situation because they don't know what to do. They did not allow themselves to entertain the idea that something bad could happen. There's no point in arguing with people that have their minds made up. Just like no one can convince you to change your mind about prepping if that's what you feel you should do.

Let's look at life in general. How many really difficult, sad, and scary situations have you been though in your life? Maybe a loved one died suddenly. Maybe you or someone you loved found out they had a life altering disease. Maybe you lost a child. Maybe you were abused. Maybe you ran into legal trouble, lost a job, or were badly injured. There are hundreds of other difficult situations that, way back when you were a child or teen, you never would have thought you would've had to experience. That's life. Always expect the unexpected and be willing to roll with the situations that come up.

I am going to pull out my Zen on you now: "That which you resist, persists." The more resistance you put up to something, the more difficult it will be for you. And resistance always comes from fear. It's fine to have opinions, but keeping an open mind to the possibility of all things helps prevent resistance.

A positive mental attitude and a belief that you will make it out fine is one of the best ways to cure your body without any medical help. It has worked for survivors that were in Africa and had to suffer alone. Some have recorded their experiences and have credited their mental thinking and faith as the reason for their survival. This shows the power of the mind and belief. You always have a choice with your thought patterns, no matter what.

SECTION FOUR – ATTITUDES TOWARD EBOLA

I have to get this out in the open because there is a huge elephant in the room. People are divided into three main groups when it comes to Ebola.

There is group 1, who is saying that Ebola is nothing but a staged event that poses zero threat to us. They say that the agenda for staging such an event is to mass vaccinate people with an Ebola vaccine that has not been tested for safety.

Group #2 is saying that the Ebola crisis is very real, and they have blind faith that our government and our elected and appointed officials will protect us. Relying on others, especially a government body with corporate interests, is never wise when it comes to life and death situations. The government is a body that is removed from emotions. It makes decisions based on the good of a certain percentage (generally those with wealth and power) and not individual needs. This will become blatantly clear if Ebola becomes a pandemic potential here in the United States.

The third group also believes the Ebola crisis is real, and they are freaking out. Sometimes fear can paralyze people and keep them from taking logical action. There is a saying that fear is more deadly than any pandemic. When lost in the wilderness, more people perish because they panic, than die from lack of food or water. When lost in the wilderness, the best course of action is to stay put, in one place, and relax. But this turns out to be that last thing people tend to do. In the Pine Barrens of New Jersey, numerous people have been found dead from exposure in the seemingly never-ending pine and scrub oak landscape after having run in large circles, following the same pathways until collapsing, exhausted. Many times, they have been found only a mile or two from the Garden State Parkway, a major highway. But panic led to disorientation, which led to action without thinking, and then death.

People that are prone to complete panic will be caught up in their emotions and not guided by a bigger plan. Dealing with someone in a panic situation when they are at the height of emotions is neither fun nor predictable.

People that are ruled by fear are also very prone to be easily influenced. We've already witness the destruction of community and unity because of the "report your neighbor" campaign. A neighbor you have barbecued with for years may see you sneeze from seasonal allergies and call 911 (or a designated number) to report that you are showing signs of Ebola because he is in so much fear of contracting the virus. It's not a good situation.

I fall somewhere in between all of them. Okay, maybe not number 2. I definitely do not believe that we should place blind faith in our government and elected and appointed officials but definitely the first and third camp.

Concerning the government, I think that we have willingly handed over our sovereignty and dignity to a ruthless corporation that is called our government. If someone comes to your door saying "I'm from the government, and I'm here to help you," would you believe them? I don't think that they took our sovereignty from us or forcibly took our constitutional rights away. I think they poked and prodded where they could, testing the waters to see where they could get control, and we willingly gave it to them.

Why?

Because it seemed easier at the time. We didn't want to take responsibility for our own actions. We invited them into our beds and then we got angry when they began to kick us out of our own bedrooms. We now see the breakdown of all of our constitutional rights[61] because things didn't fit into our individual and varied social agendas.

The Ebola Agenda

Concerning the first camp of people that says that Ebola is being used as a scare tactic to further an agenda of mass vaccinations, there is substantial evidence to suggest that Ebola may be being presented to be much worse than it actually is. There are some people, considered by many to credible, saying to be worried, while equally credible people are saying that there is nothing to worry about.

There are videos up on YouTube that allegedly show "behind the scenes" footage shot by CNN and the New York Times that document African people being paid to "act" as Ebola victims for their news releases. [62] There are other videos that outline how the government and the CDC have planned for the Ebola outbreak within the USA, long before it was even here[63]. These are just a few of the videos that seem to document this position.

If you go through the ClinicalTrials.gov website you will see in trial NCT02041715[64] that the US Government and Tekmira Pharmaceuticals Corporation have been using humans to conduct Ebola tests.

From the trial, it reads that people were given an infusion of the now famous TKM-Ebola (TKM-10080) after being exposed to the engineered Ebola virus. The trials began in January 9, 2014 and in March 2014 this new viral Ebola strain appeared in West Africa. TKM-Ebola was used to treat American Dr. Rick Sacra the first week in September.

---

61 http://www.washingtonsblog.com/2013/02/constitution.html

62 https://www.youtube.com/watch?v=-z9YuHaKr8U

63 https://www.youtube.com/watch?v=kMVlWkx-eVc

64 http://clinicaltrials.gov/show/NCT02041715

Who Owns the Ebola Virus?

Along those same lines, there is an Ebola strain that was patented in 2009. Who holds the patent? The United States government[65]. Read the summary of the invention and you will find that in 2007, the CDC was given this particular strain. It also states that the CDC holds ownership over ALL Ebola strains that show at least a 70% similarity to this created Ebola strain that has been patented. Here is the specific language from the patent itself that talks about this: *"a nucleotide sequence that has at least 70%, 75%, 80%, 85%, 90%, 95%, 96%, 97%, 98%, or 99% identity to the SEQ ID NO: 10."*

Why would the CDC claim ownership over essentially all Ebola strains?

The patent also states that a vaccine had been created at the time of the patent as well:

> *"The invention also provides kits containing compositions and formulations of the present invention. Thus, in another aspect, the invention provides a kit comprising a container containing the inventive immunogenic formulation described above. In another aspect, the invention provides a kit comprising a container containing the inventive vaccine formulation described above. "*

And,

> *"In another aspect, the invention provides vaccine preparations, including the inventive hEbola virus, including recombinant and chimeric forms of the virus, nucleic acid molecules comprised by the virus, or protein subunits of the virus. In one embodiment, the vaccine preparations of the present invention includes live but attenuated hEbola virus with or without pharmaceutically acceptable carriers, including adjuvants. In another, the vaccine preparations of the invention comprise an inactivated or killed hEbola EboBun virus, EboIC virus, or a combination thereof, with or without pharmaceutically acceptable carriers, including adjuvants. Such attenuated or inactivated viruses may be prepared by a series of passages of the virus through the host cells or by*

---

65 http://www.google.com/patents/US20120251502

preparing recombinant or chimeric forms of virus. Accordingly, the present invention further provides methods of preparing recombinant or chimeric forms of the inventive hEbola viruses described herein."

Here is where we may have the answer about why the CDC wants to hold the patent rights over all Ebola strains… because it has a primary agenda of promoting vaccines and mass vaccinations. Bill Gates, who is one of the primary faces behind the mass vaccine agenda, has donated $50,000 to the Ebola effort. Bill Gates openly talks about population control through sterilization and vaccines.[66]

Malthus Meets Monsanto

You can dress up Bill Gates and eugenics any way that you want, but the fact remains that Planned Parenthood is an offshoot of the Eugenics movement which found its rise from Malthusian-economics[67], which was one of the main inspirations for Hitler's eugenics mindset. In the video featuring Bill Gates, referenced above, you can see the connection between Bill Gates and Planned Parenthood. Monsanto, the company which has been kicked out of a number of countries due to their unwanted genetically modified foods, has also entered into the Ebola picture.[68]

Personally, any time I see Bill Gates, Monsanto, Pharmaceutical corporations and the CDC working together, I get an unsettled feeling in my stomach; especially given the possibility (or should I say probability) that there are hidden agendas and a high-level manipulation of the facts in order to meet an end.

Of course, anyone that wants to hold on to their beliefs can find fault in these videos referenced as documentation. However, it is important to keep an open mind. Could it be possible, even a tiny bit possible, that things are not as they seem? As history has shown, sometimes the truth is worse than fiction.

Ultimately, this so-called "conspiracy" scenario may or may not be true.

---

66 https://www.youtube.com/watch?v=3TyAJZVARPw

67 http://www.forbes.com/2008/12/24/malthus-dickens-scrooge-oped-cx_jb_1224bowyer.html

68 http://www.tekmira.com/partners/partnerships.php

In the big picture it doesn't really matter, as I will explain in a minute.

The last scenario is that Ebola truly is worse than we can even imagine. I am not freaking out about Ebola but I am actively concerned about the potential of this virus. I remain vigilant about the possibility of a pandemic wiping out a large number of our population all over the planet. The history of plagues is not a pretty one and there is no reason to believe that we cannot be hit with something that can cause death in a large amount of the population.[69]

More and more theories are coming out about the possibility of the Ebola virus mutating on its own. Dr. Peter Jahrling is one of the top virus scientists, and is responsible for discovering the Reston Ebola virus. Jahrling has committed his life to understanding the most dangerous viruses known to man. He has a concern that the virus may be mutating already. In his experience when you see viral loads very high, very quickly, this means a mutation in the virus.[70]

Anthony Banbury, the United Nation's top Ebola virus expert, is saying that the Ebola virus could mutate because it is fast-moving and fast-spreading. He is concerned because the more time the virus is spreading, the more chance it has to mutate.[71]

Dr. Tevin Troy, former UN secretary of human health and resources says that the Ebola virus has already mutated over 200 times. The concern is that it could go full out airborne or it could mutate enough to make its transmission more efficient.

Ultimately, the validity of any of these scenarios really does not matter. It's like theorizing about why something happened instead of concentrating on taking action. Theories won't help you, but action will. You can spend all day, every day for the rest of your life theorizing about strategies to make a million dollars, but if you do not put any ideas into action, you will die broke. All that truly matters is taking action and getting results.

69 http://uhavax.hartford.edu/bugl/histepi.htm

70 http://www.vox.com/2014/10/13/6959087/ebola-outbreak-virus-mutated-airborne

71 http://video.foxbusiness.com/v/3820245584001/former-hhs-deputy-secretary-ebola-is-definitely-mutating/#sp=show-clips

When it comes to Ebola or any other pandemic, you want a strong body. A strong body protects against infection and disease.[72] [73]

The Vaccine Debate

There is a continual, heated debate when it comes to vaccines. Many believe that vaccines have eliminated dreaded diseases like polio, smallpox, and measles. Others point out that there is substantial evidence that the vaccinations had little or nothing to do with the reduced instances of these diseases.

No matter which side of the fence you find yourself on, there is one statement that is backed by facts: Vaccines are dangerous. This has been proven over and over again in study after study, as you will read below. Whether it is an Ebola vaccine or another pandemic against which the government wants you vaccinated, a vaccine (especially a vaccine containing harmful adjuvants) shouldn't be needed if your immune system is healthy.

There is not one reputable doctor who has studied the mountains of evidence available who will say that vaccines are safe. I personally know and have worked with doctors who will not vaccinate their loved ones. Why? Because, in their opinion, the risk is too great. Medical science has no way to accurately measure the health of an immune system to know in advance if someone is susceptible to vaccine injuries.

The following is taken from the CDC website:

---Begin quote from CDC website -----------

"Common substances found in vaccines include:

Aluminum gels or salts of aluminum which are added as adjuvants to help the vaccine stimulate a better response. Adjuvants help promote an earlier, more potent response, and more persistent immune response to the vaccine.

Antibiotics which are added to some vaccines to prevent the growth of

---

72 http://www.health.harvard.edu/flu-resource-center/how-to-boost-your-immune-system.htm
73 http://www.pnas.org/content/98/13/7461.full

germs (bacteria) during production and storage of the vaccine. No vaccine produced in the United States contains penicillin.

Egg protein is found in influenza and yellow fever vaccines, which are prepared using chicken eggs. Ordinarily, persons who are able to eat eggs or egg products safely can receive these vaccines.

Formaldehyde is used to inactivate bacterial products for toxoid vaccines, (these are vaccines that use an inactive bacterial toxin to produce immunity.) It is also used to kill unwanted viruses and bacteria that might contaminate the vaccine during production. Most formaldehyde is removed from the vaccine before it is packaged.

Monosodium glutamate (MSG) and 2-phenoxy-ethanol which are used as stabilizers in a few vaccines to help the vaccine remain unchanged when the vaccine is exposed to heat, light, acidity, or humidity.

Thimerosal is a mercury-containing preservative that is added to vials of vaccine containing more than one dose in order to prevent contamination and growth of potentially harmful bacteria."

-------------------- End Quote from CDC website---

Let's take a few minutes and look a little deeper into each of these ingredients commonly used in vaccines:

Aluminum: Aluminum salts given in shots have shown to contain 1.25 mg of aluminum, which contributes to the body burden.[74] Evidence has shown that aluminum is carried to certain parts of the body including the brain[75] and lymph nodes.[76]

The body burden for aluminum is found by the total atoms of aluminum introduced into the body at one time. No human exposure

---

74 Exley C, Swarbrick L, Gherardi RK, Authier FJ: A role for the body burden of aluminium in vaccine-associated macrophagic myofasciitis and chronic fatigue syndrome. Med Hyp 2009

75 Khan Z, Combadière C, Authier FJ, Itier V, Lux F, Exley C, Mahrouf-Yorgov M, Decrouy X, Moretto P, Tillement O, Gherardi RK, Cadusseau J: Slow CCL2-dependent translocation of bio persistent particles from muscle to brain. BMC Med J 2013

76 Gheradi RK, Coquet M, Cherin P, Belec L, Moretto P, Dreyfuss PA, Pellissier JF, Chariot P, Authier FJ: Macrophagic myofasciitis lesions assess long-term persistence of vaccine-derived aluminium hydroxide in muscle. Brain 2001

to aluminum is safe or innocuous.[77] [78] Exposure to aluminum from health products, grooming products, environmental exposure, and food exposure[79] cause aluminum toxicity due to build-up.

Aluminum toxicity has shown to be linked to chronic fatigue, autoimmune disease, autism, gulf war syndrome, multiple sclerosis, seizures, thyroid problems, and neurological disorders and diseases.[80]

Antibiotics: While I understand the reasoning behind the inclusion of antibiotics in vaccines, it does not make it good for the body. Antibiotics will wipe out the natural good flora in your body. Guess what? A big part of your immune system is healthy flora.[81] If that is diminished or wiped out, then you have a lower natural immune resistance to infective viruses and bacteria.[82]

Antibiotics have shown to have a long term effect, not just an isolated short term impact. Antibiotic resistant strains can then live and thrive in your inner ecology making you more susceptible to illness.[83]

Egg Protein: Often used to grow viruses for vaccines, chicken eggs are only one source of medium for growth. Others include monkey cells, human cells, and genetically modified organisms.[84] While it is believed that none of these pose a risk to vaccinated individuals, one of the biggest scandals around vaccinations involved the polio vaccine, which was grown on monkey tissue infected with the SV40 virus. While the CDC initially admitted that as many as 30 million Americans could be at risk for cancer due to the polio vaccine,[85] they later removed pages from their website that provided information about the

---

77 Exley C: Human exposure to aluminium. Env Sci: Process Impacts 2013, 15:1807-1816

78 EFSA: On the evaluation of a new study related to the bioavailability of aluminium in food. EFSA J 2011

79 Pali-Schöll I, Jensen-Jarolim E: Anti-acid medication as a risk factor for food allergy. Allergy 2011

80 Tomljenovic L, Shaw CA: Aluminum vaccine adjuvants: are they safe? Curr Med Chem 2011

81 Fuller, R. and Perdigon, G. Gut Flora, Nutrition, Immunity and Health. Blackwell Publishing, 2003.

82 Rebeca Martín, Sylvie Miquel, Jonathan Ulmer, Noura Kechaou, Philippe Langella, et al. Role of commensal and probiotic bacteria in human health: a focus on inflammatory bowel disease. Microbial Cell Factories 2013

83 Cecilia Jernberg, Sonja Löfmark,,Charlotta Edlund and Janet K. Jansson. Long-term impacts of antibiotic exposure on the human intestinal microbiota. Microbiology, 2010.

84 http://www.ovg.ox.ac.uk/vaccine-ingredients#human-cell-lines

85 http://www.thelibertybeacon.com/2013/07/12/cdc-admits-as-many-as-30-million-americans-could-be-at-risk-for-cancer-due-to-polio-vaccine/

connection.[86] However archived versions of the pages are available. [87,88]

This vaccine not only caused polio in many recipients, it killed many hundreds. It is also believed that the polio vaccine, administered to nearly one hundred million people worldwide, could be the direct cause of a huge spike in soft tissue cancers, as discussed above. In addition, there is a substantial body of evidence suggesting that the virtual elimination of polio had nothing to do with vaccines.[89]

Formaldehyde: The government declared formaldehyde a known cancer causing agent in June 2010, so I am unsure why it is considered safe in vaccinations. Formaldehyde is an embalming fluid which helps to keep body tissues firm.

Again, from the CDC website: "Formaldehyde exposure is a special concern for children and the elderly. Children may become sensitive to formaldehyde more easily, which may make it more likely they will become sick."[90]

Formaldehyde damage was once thought to be reversible. However, more recent research shows that formaldehyde can be distributed enough throughout the DNA to damage it irreversibly.[91]

Monosodium glutamate (MSG): Typically a food additive that many experts warn people to avoid. MSG has been shown to have neurotoxic effects. It is also an excitotoxin, causes metabolic effects,[92] and can lead to obesity.[93] MSG causes changes in the prefrontal area of the brain, brain cell death, shrinking of the pituitary, and leads to fewer viable neurons. As my son likes to say, MSG will poke holes in your brain and

---

86 http://www.medicaldaily.com/cdc-removes-webpage-about-polio-vaccine-contamination-further-admission-guilt-249339

87https://web.archive.org/web/20100308102630/http://www.cdc.gov/vaccinesafety/updates/archive/polio_and_cancer.htm

88https://web.archive.org/web/20110307094146/http://www.cdc.gov/vaccinesafety/updates/archive/polio_and_cancer_factsheet.htm

89For example: http://www.rense.com/general92/polio.htm

90 www.cdc.gov/nceh/drywall/docs/whatyoushouldknowaboutformaldehyde.pdf

91 Carolyn J. Collins and Walter R. Guild. Irreversible effects of formaldehyde on DNA. Science Direct.

92 Afifi, M. M. & Abbas, A. M. (2011). "Monosodium Glutamate versus Diet Induced Obesity in Pregnant Rats and Their Offspring," Acta Physiologica Hungarica, 98(2), 177-88.

93 http://articles.mercola.com/sites/articles/archive/2009/04/21/msg-is-this-silent-killer-lurking-in-your-kitchen-cabinets.aspx

make you fat.

Thimerosal. Thimerosal is a mercury-containing preservative. Remember how mercury was banned from being used in thermometers because of its toxicity? But yet we should believe that it is okay to inject into our bodies as long as it's in a vaccine. There are hundreds of other preservatives that could be used instead. Look at our food system, the preservatives in there can yield a shelf life of up to 20 years with some products. Surely there is something safer to use as a preservative. Even in small doses, mercury should be avoided.

Looking at the multitude of research papers proving the dangers of thimerosal, it is mind boggling how this is allowed to be put into vaccinations. Even the CDC, on its website, states that in July 1999, the Public Health Service agencies, the American Academy of Pediatrics, and even vaccine manufacturers themselves all agreed that thimerosol should be reduced or eliminated in vaccines "as a precautionary measure."[94]

And, yes, even though the manufacturers eliminated thimerosol from most vaccines, they still put it into some, including the influenza vaccine. And, even after 1999, the CDC continued to release study after study allegedly "proving" that vaccines containing thimerosol were safe. But there is more to the story, as you'll discover below.

But first, here are just a few of the problems associated with thimerosol:

Thimerosal disperses quickly to the vital organs of the body, especially the brain and kidneys.[95] Once there, it begins to release mercury gas.[96]

Cells begin to kill themselves[97] and DNA breakage[98] has been observed

94 http://www.cdc.gov/vaccinesafety/Concerns/thimerosal/thimerosal_timeline.html

95 Magos, L., Brown, A. W., Sparrow, S., Bailey, E., Snowden, R. T., and Skipp, W. R. (1985). The comparative toxicology of ethyl- and methylmercury. Arch. Toxicol. 57, 260–267

96 Blair, A., Clark, B., Clarke, A., and Wood, P. (1975). Tissue concentrations of mercury after chronic dosing of squirrel monkeys with thimerosal. Toxicology 3, 171–176.

97 Makani, S., Gollapudi, S., Yel, L., Chiplunkar, S., and Gupta, S. (2002). Biochemical and molecular basis of thimerosal-induced apoptosis in T-cells: Major role of mitochondrial pathway. Genes Immun. 3, 270–278.

98 Baskin, D. S., Ngo, H., and Didenko, V. V. (2003). Thimerosal induces DNA breaks, caspase-3 activation, membrane

when thimerosal is introduced into the body.

That's not all the damage that thimerosal causes. A scientific paper regarding thimerosol in vaccines was peer-reviewed, approved, and then published in June of 2014. This paper pointed out that over 165 different studies[99] conducted over a 75-year period had proved and documented dangers from thimerosol and thimerosol-containing vaccines.

The dangers and consequences included ADHD, autism, acrodynia, allergic reactions, autoimmune reactions, death, developmental delays in children, neuro-developmental disorders, delay in speaking, poisoning, malformations, tics, and Well's syndrome.[100, 101]

The paper then focused in detail on 6 particular studies, funded by the CDC. These are studies which the agency has used repeatedly to bolster their claim that thimerosol is safe, and that there is no correlation between autism and administration of vaccines, especially in the face of published outcomes of non-CDC-funded studies over a 75-year period.

The conclusion of this paper was that the CDC had purposely omitted any data that might have been harmful to the agency's agenda of mass vaccination, and the CDC had knowingly ignored almost eight decades of data in direct conflict with their position of "thimerosol is safe in vaccines for children."

I really could go on and on about the damage that thimerosal does to the body, brain, and nervous system but I'm sure you get the point.

It's not that I am completely against vaccines, even though I had a son that was injured by the MMR vaccine. I believe in the principal of vaccines. The principal is: "Like cures like," which is based on a

---

damage and cell death in cultured human neurons and fibroblasts. Toxicol. Sci. 74, 361–368

99 For a comprehensive list of the 165+ studies, follow this link: http://mercury-freedrugs.org/docs/20140329_Kern_JK_ExcelFile_TM_sHarm_ReferenceList_v33.xlsx

100 Brian Hooker, Janet Kern, David Geier, Boyd Haley, Lisa Sykes, Paul King, and Mark Geier. Methodological Issues and Evidence of Malfeasance in Research Purporting to Show Thimerosal in Vaccines Is Safe. BioMed Research International. 2012.

101 To read the entire peer-reviewed and published paper, go to this link: http://www.hindawi.com/journals/bmri/2014/247218/

foundational rule of homeopathy. Of course, most mainstream medical professionals consider homeopathic medicine to be quackery, even while this is the principal upon which the entire vaccination program is based. What have become dangerous are not necessarily the active components in the vaccines themselves, but the myriad additives, adjuvants, and growth mediums that can not only tear down the immune system but poison the body as well. Unfortunately, some of that damage will not be seen until years down the road.

When my son was injured by the MMR vaccine, I found out that I wasn't alone... not by a long shot. In fact, the government has created The Vaccine Injury Act[102] and the National Vaccine Injury Compensation Act[103] in order to compensate injured recipients of vaccines. They knew that these injuries were inevitable, and set up funds for the inevitable lawsuits. Why else would these Acts have been passed and money set aside to compensate victims?

Regarding the June, 2014 paper uncovering the blatant and persistent wrong doing of the CDC, here is a brief quote:

"Dr. Boyd Haley, international expert in mercury toxicity and a co-author of the recently published paper said "There is no doubt that authorities in the CDC have initiated and participated in a cover-up of vaccine-induced damage from thimerosal to our children—-and this I consider criminal." The paper, "Methodological Issues and Evidence of Malfeasance in Research Purporting to Show Thimerosal in Vaccines is Safe"[104] was published on June 6 and contains eight pages of evidence that the CDC has had knowledge of the vaccine preservative's neurological risks, yet continues to cover them up.

The paper concludes, "five of the publications examined in this review were directly commissioned by the CDC, raising the possible issue of conflict of interests or research bias, since vaccine promotion is a central mission of the CDC. Conceivably, if serious neurological disorders are found to be related to thimerosal in vaccines, such findings could possibly be viewed as damaging to the vaccine program."

Dr. Hooker has submitted over 100 FOIA requests to the CDC over the past 10

---

102 http://www.nap.edu/openbook.php?record_id=12796&page=243

103 http://www.hrsa.gov/vaccinecompensation/index.html

104 http://www.hindawi.com/journals/bmri/2014/247218/

years and has amassed thousands of pages of documents showing malfeasance in the CDC's vaccine safety program. Hooker revealed that one CDC document quoted a top official instructing CDC employees to "Review all correspondences and documents to see if there is 'foreseeable harm' to the agency if they were released" so the documents could be redacted by CDC attorneys prior to release."

I will leave you with some words from the current FBI Director, James Comey, in an interview he did with 60 Minutes which aired on October 5th of 2014.[105] At the 00:47 mark, he says, **"Americans should be deeply skeptical of government power. You cannot trust people in power. Our founders knew that…"**

If you are interested in knowing how to combat the effects of vaccination in the case that you are force vaccinated, you can download an effective protocol at: http://www.ScrewEbola.com/combat

105 http://www.againstcronycapitalism.org/2014/10/fbi-director-james-comey-on-60-minutes-americans-should-be-deeply-skeptical-of-government-power-video/

SECTION FIVE – IN CONCLUSION

There is not much more to say about the current Ebola crisis. I do feel that we may be in for a bumpy ride, despite the lull in any confirmed Ebola cases. We could well be in the middle of the calm before the storm.

Never has there been a time in history where our officials have gone to great lengths to follow through on the speculation of pandemic diseases. There have always been announcements on how to deal with pandemic situations but nothing really moved forward. Now, things have moved forward and continue to move forward with the following announcements:

- A newly formed CDC SWAT team.[106]
- The October 20, 2014 Pentagon appointed "strike team" that consists of 30 specialized trained military personnel to stay within the USA borders and react to an Ebola crisis.[107]
- The October 22nd announcement that the 'state-of-the-art' Bio-Containment Facilities in Texas are now ready for Texans that have Ebola.[108]
- The appointment of Ron Klain as the Ebola Czar.[109]

---

106 http://abcnews.go.com/Health/wireStory/cdc-details-ebola-response-prep-teams-26403021

107 http://www.cnn.com/2014/10/19/health/us-ebola/index.html

108 http://governor.state.tx.us/news/press-release/20256/

109http://www.forbes.com/sites/steveforbes/2014/10/19/obamas-ebola-czar-is-a-dangerous-mistake-here-are-3-who-could-do-the-job/

It is interesting that a state-of-the-art Bio Containment facility has been specially designed and outfitted with the CDC and a few local hospitals in a matter of a few weeks.

Remember, it was repeatedly told to everyone through to the end of September that Ebola would not come here. I'm not sure about you but I don't think I've ever witnessed anything in government or hospital politics moving this quickly. Heck, there isn't any construction in Texas that moves quickly. Since one of the locations, the Methodist Campus for Continuing Care in Richardson, Texas had been vacant for quite a long time, renovation prior to October 1st would probably go unnoticed.

For updates and breaking news about Ebola, please visit http://www.ScrewEbola.com, where you will also find alternatives to vaccines, how to make your own vaccines for Ebola or any other pandemic, as well as the detox protocol mentioned above.

In addition, you'll find links to resources for everything you might need during this difficult time.

If you want to know what specific products I am personally using for myself and my family, type the following link into any web browser:

http://astore.amazon.com/ebola_protocol-20

For ongoing updates, vaccine detox protocols, resource guides, and homemade vaccine techniques and documentation, visit:

www.ScrewEbola.com

ABOUT THE AUTHOR

Wilton M. Evans is a twenty-year student of health and wellness along with individual freedom and personal responsibility. His fascination with how the human body works led him to a career providing alternative treatments for clients dissatisfied with the status quo. He is a frequent traveler, and lives in Dallas with his wife and two children.